Welcome to the **"Carnivore Diet Cookbook for Seniors: Transform Your Diet with Protein-Rich, Senior-Friendly Recipes."** This cookbook is designed specifically for seniors who are seeking to enhance their health and vitality through a nourishing, meat-focused diet. Whether you are new to the carnivore lifestyle or looking to expand your culinary repertoire, this book is your gateway to discovering the numerous benefits of a protein-rich diet.

As we age, our nutritional needs change. Maintaining muscle mass, bone density, and overall energy levels becomes increasingly important. A diet rich in high-quality animal proteins can play a significant role in supporting these health goals. The carnivore diet, which emphasizes meat, fish, and animal-based products, is known for its simplicity and nutrient density, making it an ideal choice for seniors looking to optimize their well-being.

In this cookbook, you will find over 110 delicious and easy-to-prepare recipes that cater to the unique dietary needs of seniors. From hearty breakfasts and satisfying lunches to savory dinners and delightful snacks, each recipe is crafted to provide the essential nutrients your body needs to thrive. Our recipes focus on whole, natural ingredients and are free from processed foods and unnecessary additives, ensuring that you get the purest form of nutrition.

The journey to better health starts with making informed choices about what you eat. By incorporating these protein-rich, senior-friendly recipes into your daily routine, you can experience improved energy levels, enhanced mental clarity, and better overall health. Whether you're looking to lose weight, gain strength, or simply enjoy delicious meals, this cookbook offers a variety of options to suit your tastes and health goals.

We understand that cooking can sometimes be a daunting task, especially if you're adjusting to a new dietary lifestyle. That's why we've included helpful tips, cooking techniques, and nutritional information to guide you along the way. Our goal is to make your transition to the carnivore diet as smooth and enjoyable as possible.

Embark on this culinary adventure with us and discover how the carnivore diet can transform your health and well-being. Here's to a healthier, more vibrant you!

1. Scrambled eggs with bacon

Ingredient:

- 6 large eggs
- 2 tablespoons milk or cream
- 1/4 teaspoon salt
- 1/8 teaspoon black pepper
- 4 slices bacon, cooked until crispy and crumbled

Instructions:

1. In a medium bowl, whisk together the eggs, milk/cream, salt, and pepper until well combined.

2. Cook the bacon in a skillet over medium heat until crispy. Remove the bacon from the skillet and crumble it.

3. Pour the egg mixture into the same skillet with the bacon drippings. Use a spatula to gently push the eggs from the edge of the pan towards the center as they cook, creating soft, fluffy curds.

4. Continue cooking the eggs, stirring occasionally, until they are softly scrambled, about 2•3 minutes total.

5. Remove the scrambled eggs from the heat and stir in the crumbled bacon.

6. Serve the scrambled eggs with bacon immediately, while hot. Enjoy!

2. Omelette with cheese and ham

Ingredient:

- 3 large eggs
- 2 tablespoons butter or ghee
- 2 ounces shredded cheddar cheese
- 2 ounces diced ham

Instructions:

1. Crack the eggs into a small bowl and beat them lightly with a fork until well combined.

2. Melt the butter or ghee in a small non•stick skillet over medium heat.

3. Pour the beaten eggs into the skillet and let them sit for 20•30 seconds to set the bottom.

4. Using a spatula, gently push the cooked egg from the edges towards the center, tilting the pan to allow the uncooked egg to flow to the edges. Do this all the way around the pan.

5. Once the eggs are mostly set but still a bit runny on top, sprinkle the shredded cheddar cheese and diced ham evenly over half of the omelette.

6. Use the spatula to fold the unfilled half of the omelette over the filled half.

7. Slide the omelette onto a plate and serve immediately.

This omelette is perfect for a carnivore diet, as it's high in protein from the eggs and ham, and contains only animal•based ingredients. Enjoy!

3. Steak and eggs

Ingredient:

- 1 (8-10 oz) ribeye steak, about 1-inch thick
- 2 tablespoons olive oil or butter
- 2 large eggs
- Salt and pepper to taste

Instructions:

1. Pat the steak dry with paper towels and season generously with salt and pepper on both sides.

2. Heat a cast-iron skillet or heavy-bottomed pan over high heat. Add the olive oil or butter and swirl to coat the pan.

3. When the pan is very hot, add the steak. Cook for 3-4 minutes per side for medium-rare, or until it reaches your desired doneness. Transfer the steak to a plate and let it rest for 5 minutes.

4. Reduce the heat to medium and crack the eggs directly into the hot pan. Cook the eggs to your desired doneness, about 2-3 minutes for sunny-side up or 4-5 minutes for over-easy.

5. Slice the steak against the grain and serve it immediately alongside the fried eggs.

6. Season the eggs with additional salt and pepper if desired.

This simple steak and eggs dish is a classic carnivore-friendly meal that's high in protein and nutrients. The juicy steak pairs perfectly with the runny yolks of the fried eggs. Enjoy!

4. Sausage patties

Ingredient:

- 1 lb ground pork
- 1 tsp salt
- 1 tsp black pepper
- 1 tsp dried sage
- 1/2 tsp dried thyme
- 1/4 tsp cayenne pepper (optional)

Instructions:

1. In a large bowl, combine the ground pork, salt, black pepper, dried sage, dried thyme, and cayenne pepper (if using). Mix well until the seasonings are evenly distributed.

2. Divide the seasoned pork into 8 equal portions. Roll each portion into a ball, then flatten it into a patty about 1/2•inch thick.

3. Heat a large skillet or griddle over medium•high heat. Add the sausage patties in a single layer, being careful not to overcrowd the pan.

4. Cook the sausage patties for 3•4 minutes per side, or until they are cooked through and browned on both sides. The internal temperature should reach 160°F.

5. Transfer the cooked sausage patties to a paper towel•lined plate to drain any excess fat.

6. Serve the sausage patties warm, either on their own or as part of a larger carnivore•friendly breakfast.

These homemade sausage patties are perfect for a carnivore diet. You can adjust the seasonings to your taste, and they pair well with eggs, cheese, or other carnivore•friendly ingredients.

5. Pork belly slices

Ingredient:

- 1 lb pork belly, skin on and cut into 1/2•inch thick slices
- 1 tsp salt
- 1/2 tsp black pepper
- 1 tsp baking soda

Instructions:

1. Pat the pork belly slices dry with paper towels and place them on a baking sheet. Sprinkle the salt, pepper, and baking soda evenly over the top of the pork belly slices.

2. Refrigerate the pork belly slices uncovered for at least 2 hours, or up to 24 hours. This will help dry out the skin and create a crispy texture.

3. Preheat your oven to 400°F (200°C).

4. Line a baking sheet with parchment paper or a silicone baking mat. Arrange the pork belly slices in a single layer on the prepared baking sheet.

5. Roast the pork belly slices for 30•40 minutes, flipping them halfway through, until the skin is crispy and golden brown.

6. For extra crispiness, you can broil the pork belly slices for 2•3 minutes at the end, watching carefully to prevent burning.

7. Remove the pork belly slices from the oven and let them rest for 5 minutes before serving.

These crispy pork belly slices are perfect for a carnivore diet. Serve them on their own as a main dish, or use them in other recipes like salads, stir•fries, or as a topping for eggs.

Enjoy your delicious pork belly!

6. Beef liver and eggs

Ingredient:

- 1 lb beef liver, sliced into 1/4•inch thick pieces
- 4 tablespoons butter or ghee, divided
- 6 large eggs
- Salt and pepper to taste

Instructions:

1. Pat the beef liver slices dry with paper towels and season them generously with salt and pepper on both sides.

2. In a large skillet, melt 2 tablespoons of the butter or ghee over medium•high heat. Working in batches if needed, add the liver slices in a single layer and cook for 2•3 minutes per side, until browned on the outside but still slightly pink in the center. Transfer the cooked liver to a plate and set aside.

3. In the same skillet, melt the remaining 2 tablespoons of butter or ghee over medium heat. Crack the eggs directly into the pan and cook them to your desired doneness, about 2•3 minutes for sunny•side up or 4•5 minutes for over•easy.

4. Serve the fried eggs immediately, topped with the seared beef liver slices. Season with additional salt and pepper if desired.

This beef liver and eggs dish is a nutrient•dense, carnivore•friendly meal that's high in protein, iron, and other essential vitamins and minerals. The combination of the tender, flavorful liver and the runny egg yolks is simply delicious.

7. Fried eggs in butter

Ingredient:

- 2 tablespoons unsalted butter
- 4 large eggs
- Salt and pepper to taste

Instructions:

1. In a non•stick skillet, melt the butter over medium heat. Make sure the butter coats the entire surface of the pan.

2. Crack the eggs directly into the hot, buttered skillet. Be careful not to overcrowd the pan • you may need to cook the eggs in batches.

3. Cook the eggs for 2•3 minutes, or until the whites are completely set but the yolks are still runny.

4. Season the fried eggs with salt and pepper to taste.

5. Carefully transfer the fried eggs to a plate and serve immediately.

Tips:
- For best results, use fresh, high•quality eggs.

- Basting the eggs with the hot butter during cooking can help the whites set while keeping the yolks runny.

- You can also cover the pan with a lid for the last minute of cooking to help the whites set.

- Adjust the heat as needed to prevent the butter from burning.

These simple fried eggs in butter are a perfect carnivore•friendly breakfast or snack. The rich, creamy yolks pair perfectly with the nutty, browned butter. Enjoy!

8. Eggs Benedict with hollandaise sauce (no bread)

Ingredient:

For the Hollandaise Sauce:
- 3 egg yolks
- 1/2 cup (1 stick) unsalted butter, melted
- 1 tbsp lemon juice
- 1/4 tsp salt
- Pinch of cayenne pepper (optional)

For the Eggs Benedict:
- 4 eggs
- 4 slices Canadian bacon or ham
- 2 tbsp white vinegar

Instructions:

1. Make the Hollandaise Sauce:
   - In a medium bowl, whisk the egg yolks until they are thick and pale yellow.
   - Slowly drizzle in the melted butter while whisking constantly until the sauce is thick and creamy.
   - Whisk in the lemon juice, salt, and cayenne pepper (if using). Keep the sauce warm.

2. Poach the Eggs:
   - Fill a large skillet with 3•4 inches of water and bring to a gentle simmer. Add the white vinegar.
   - Crack each egg individually into a small ramekin or cup, then gently slide the egg into the simmering water.
   - Poach the eggs for 4•5 minutes, until the whites are set but the yolks are still runny.
   - Remove the poached eggs from the water using a slotted spoon.

3. Assemble the Eggs Benedict:
   - Place a slice of Canadian bacon or ham on a plate.
   - Top the bacon/ham with a poached egg.
   - Drizzle the warm hollandaise sauce over the top of the egg.
   - Serve immediately.

This carnivore•friendly Eggs Benedict is a delicious and nutrient•dense breakfast or brunch option. The rich, creamy hollandaise sauce complements the runny egg yolks and savory Canadian bacon perfectly.

9. Carnivore pancakes (made with pork rinds and eggs)

Ingredient:

- 1 cup pork rinds, finely crushed into a powder
- 4 large eggs
- 1/4 cup heavy cream (or unsweetened almond milk)
- 1/2 tsp baking powder
- 1/4 tsp salt

Instructions:

1. In a medium bowl, whisk together the crushed pork rind powder, eggs, heavy cream (or almond milk), baking powder, and salt until well combined.

2. Heat a non•stick skillet or griddle over medium heat. Grease the surface with a small amount of butter or avocado oil.

3. Scoop the batter onto the hot surface, using about 2•3 tablespoons per pancake. Cook for 2•3 minutes per side, or until golden brown.

4. Flip the pancakes carefully and cook the other side until cooked through.

5. Serve the carnivore pancakes warm, with your desired toppings. Some tasty options include:
   - Fried eggs
   - Crumbled bacon or sausage
   - Shredded cheese
   - Avocado
   - Butter or ghee

These pork rind pancakes are a great low•carb, high•protein option for a carnivore diet. The pork rinds provide a nice texture and flavor, while the eggs help bind the pancakes together.

Enjoy your delicious carnivore•friendly pancakes!

10. Cream cheese omelette

Ingredient:

- 3 large eggs
- 2 tablespoons cream cheese, softened
- 1 tablespoon butter
- Salt and pepper to taste

Instructions:

1. Crack the eggs into a small bowl and beat them lightly with a fork until well combined.

2. In a separate small bowl, mix the softened cream cheese until it's smooth and creamy.

3. Melt the butter in a small non•stick skillet over medium heat.

4. Pour the beaten eggs into the hot skillet. As the eggs start to set around the edges, use a spatula to gently push the cooked egg towards the center, tilting the pan to allow the uncooked egg to flow to the edges.

5. When the eggs are mostly set but still a bit runny on top, dollop the softened cream cheese over half of the omelette.

6. Use the spatula to fold the unfilled half of the omelette over the cream cheese•filled half.

7. Slide the omelette onto a plate and serve immediately, seasoning with salt and pepper to taste.

The creamy, tangy cream cheese pairs beautifully with the fluffy eggs in this simple carnivore•friendly omelette. You can also try adding other fillings like cooked bacon, ham, or shredded cheese.

Enjoy your delicious cream cheese omelette!

11. Smoked salmon with scrambled eggs

Ingredient:

- 4 large eggs
- 2 tbsp milk
- 1 tbsp butter
- 2 oz smoked salmon, chopped
- 1 tbsp chopped fresh dill (optional)
- Salt and pepper to taste

Instructions:

1. In a small bowl, whisk together the eggs and milk until well combined.

2. Melt the butter in a non•stick skillet over medium heat.

3. Pour the egg mixture into the skillet and let it sit for 20•30 seconds to set the bottom slightly.

4. Using a spatula, gently push the eggs from the edge of the pan towards the center, tilting the pan to allow the uncooked egg to flow to the edges. Continue doing this until the eggs are softly scrambled, about 2•3 minutes total.

5. Remove the pan from the heat and stir in the chopped smoked salmon and dill (if using).

6. Season with salt and pepper to taste.

7. Serve the scrambled eggs with the smoked salmon immediately, while hot.

This makes a delicious and protein•packed breakfast or brunch dish. The smoky salmon pairs beautifully with the creamy scrambled eggs. Enjoy!

12. Cheese•stuffed sausage links

Ingredient:

- 1 lb Italian sausage links, casings removed
- 4 oz cream cheese, softened
- 1/2 cup shredded cheddar cheese
- 1 tbsp chopped fresh parsley
- 1/4 tsp garlic powder
- Salt and pepper to taste

Instructions:

1. In a medium bowl, mix together the cream cheese, cheddar cheese, parsley, garlic powder, salt, and pepper until well combined.

2. Divide the sausage meat into 8 equal portions. Flatten each portion into a thin patty.

3. Place a heaping tablespoon of the cheese mixture in the center of each sausage patty.

4. Carefully wrap the sausage around the cheese filling, sealing the edges to completely enclose the cheese.

5. Heat a large skillet over medium•high heat. Add the stuffed sausage links and cook for 4•5 minutes per side, until the sausage is cooked through and the cheese is melted.

6. Serve the cheese•stuffed sausage links hot, garnished with additional chopped parsley if desired.

These make a delicious and impressive appetizer or main dish. The melty cheese center is a tasty surprise inside the savory sausage. Enjoy!

13. Beef breakfast burrito (using cheese wrap)

Ingredient:

- 1 lb ground beef
- 1 tbsp taco seasoning
- 1/2 cup diced onion
- 1/2 cup diced bell pepper
- 6 eggs, scrambled
- 1 cup shredded cheddar cheese
- 4 low•carb or keto cheese wraps (or regular tortillas)
- Salsa, sour cream, and hot sauce for serving (optional)

Instructions:

1. In a large skillet over medium•high heat, cook the ground beef until browned and crumbled, 5•7 minutes. Drain any excess fat.

2. Add the taco seasoning, onion, and bell pepper to the skillet. Cook for 3•4 minutes until the vegetables are softened.

3. In a separate skillet, scramble the eggs until cooked through.

4. To assemble the burritos:
   - Lay a cheese wrap or tortilla flat on a work surface.
   - Spoon some of the beef mixture down the center of the wrap.
   - Top with scrambled eggs and shredded cheddar cheese.
   - Fold the bottom of the wrap up over the filling, then fold in the sides and continue rolling tightly into a burrito shape.

5. Heat a skillet or griddle over medium heat. Place the burrito seam•side down and cook for 2•3 minutes per side until lightly browned.

6. Serve the breakfast burritos warm, with salsa, sour cream, and hot sauce on the side if desired.

The cheese wrap helps hold everything together and adds extra cheesy flavor to these hearty breakfast burritos. Enjoy!

14. Bone marrow on toast (use cheese slices as toast)

Ingredient:

- 4 pieces of beef bone marrow, about 1•inch thick each
- 4 slices of cheddar or Swiss cheese
- Coarse sea salt
- Freshly ground black pepper
- Chopped parsley or chives (optional garnish)

Instructions:

1. Preheat your oven to 400°F (200°C).

2. Place the bone marrow pieces on a baking sheet or in a baking dish. Roast for 15•20 minutes, until the marrow is soft and starting to ooze out of the bones.

3. Remove the baking sheet from the oven and let the bone marrow cool slightly, about 5 minutes.

4. While the bone marrow is cooling, place the cheese slices on a separate baking sheet or in a broiler•safe dish.

5. Once the bone marrow is slightly cooled, use a spoon to scoop the soft, creamy marrow out of the bones and onto the cheese slices.

6. Place the cheese and bone marrow under the broiler for 2•3 minutes, just until the cheese is melted and starting to bubble.

7. Remove from the oven and season the bone marrow with a generous sprinkle of coarse sea salt and freshly ground black pepper.

8. Garnish with chopped parsley or chives, if desired.

9. Serve the bone marrow on cheese slices immediately, while hot.

The rich, buttery bone marrow pairs beautifully with the melted cheese, creating a decadent and flavorful open•faced "toast" or appetizer. Enjoy!

15. Ground beef and egg scramble

Ingredient:

- 1 lb ground beef
- 1 onion, diced
- 2 cloves garlic, minced
- 8 eggs
- 2 tbsp milk
- 1 tsp dried oregano
- Salt and pepper to taste
- Shredded cheddar cheese (optional)
- Chopped parsley or green onions for garnish (optional)

Instructions:

1. In a large skillet over medium•high heat, cook the ground beef, breaking it up with a spatula, until browned and cooked through, about 5•7 minutes. Drain any excess fat.

2. Add the diced onion and minced garlic to the skillet. Cook for 2•3 minutes until the onion is translucent.

3. In a medium bowl, whisk together the eggs and milk. Season with the dried oregano, salt, and pepper.

4. Pour the egg mixture into the skillet with the ground beef and onions. Use a spatula to gently scramble the eggs, stirring frequently, until the eggs are cooked through but still soft, about 3•5 minutes.

5. Remove the skillet from heat. If desired, sprinkle the scramble with shredded cheddar cheese.

6. Serve the ground beef and egg scramble hot, garnished with chopped parsley or green onions if desired.

This is a simple yet satisfying breakfast or brunch dish that combines savory ground beef, fluffy scrambled eggs, and optional melted cheese. It's a great way to start the day with protein and nutrients. Enjoy!

16. Chicken liver pâté

Ingredient:

- 1 lb chicken livers, trimmed of any connective tissue
- 1/2 cup unsalted butter, softened
- 1/4 cup heavy cream
- 2 tbsp brandy or cognac (optional)
- 1 tsp Dijon mustard
- 1 tsp fresh thyme leaves
- 1/2 tsp ground black pepper
- 1/4 tsp ground nutmeg
- 1/4 tsp salt

Instructions:

1. In a large skillet, cook the chicken livers over medium•high heat for 5•7 minutes, stirring occasionally, until they are cooked through but still slightly pink in the center. Transfer the livers to a food processor.

2. Add the softened butter, heavy cream, brandy (if using), Dijon mustard, thyme, black pepper, nutmeg, and salt to the food processor. Blend until the mixture is smooth and creamy, about 2•3 minutes, scraping down the sides as needed.

3. Transfer the pâté to a serving dish or ramekins. Cover the surface with plastic wrap or parchment paper to prevent a skin from forming.

4. Refrigerate the pâté for at least 2 hours, or up to 5 days, before serving.

5. When ready to serve, remove the pâté from the refrigerator and let it come to room temperature for 15•20 minutes.

6. Serve the chicken liver pâté with crackers, toasted bread, or crostini. Garnish with additional fresh thyme leaves if desired.

The rich, creamy pâté is delicious spread on crisp bread or crackers. The brandy and spices add depth of flavor to this classic appetizer. Enjoy!

17. Duck eggs with prosciutto

Ingredient:

- 4 duck eggs
- 2 tbsp butter
- 2 oz thinly sliced prosciutto
- Salt and pepper to taste
- Chopped chives or parsley for garnish (optional)

Instructions:

1. Crack the duck eggs into a bowl, being careful not to break the yolks.

2. In a non•stick skillet, melt the butter over medium heat.

3. Gently pour the duck eggs into the skillet. Cook for 2•3 minutes, or until the whites are set but the yolks are still runny.

4. Arrange the slices of prosciutto around the eggs in the skillet.

5. Season the duck eggs with salt and pepper to taste.

6. Carefully transfer the duck eggs and prosciutto to plates.

7. Garnish with chopped chives or parsley, if desired.

Serve the duck eggs with prosciutto immediately, while hot.

The rich, creamy duck eggs pair beautifully with the salty, savory prosciutto. The runny yolks create a delicious sauce when broken. This makes a luxurious and protein•packed breakfast or brunch dish.

Duck eggs have a richer, creamier texture compared to chicken eggs, which makes them perfect for this simple yet elegant preparation. Enjoy!

18. Lamb chops and eggs

Ingredient:

- 4 lamb chops, about 1•inch thick
- 2 tbsp olive oil
- Salt and pepper to taste
- 4 eggs
- 2 tbsp butter
- Chopped parsley for garnish (optional)

Instructions:

1. Season the lamb chops generously with salt and pepper on both sides.

2. Heat a large skillet or grill pan over medium•high heat. Add the olive oil.

3. When the oil is hot, add the lamb chops and cook for 3•4 minutes per side for medium•rare, or until they reach your desired doneness. Transfer the cooked chops to a plate and let them rest.

4. In the same skillet, melt the butter over medium heat.

5. Crack the eggs directly into the skillet and cook for 2•3 minutes for sunny•side up, or until the whites are set but the yolks are still runny.

6. Serve the lamb chops immediately, topped with the fried eggs. Garnish with chopped parsley if desired.

You can also prepare the eggs in any other style you prefer, such as over•easy, over•medium, or scrambled.

The rich, flavorful lamb pairs beautifully with the runny egg yolks for a delicious and protein•packed meal. Enjoy this simple yet elegant dish!

19. Turkey bacon and eggs

Ingredient:

- 6 slices turkey bacon
- 4 large eggs
- 1 tbsp butter
- Salt and pepper to taste
- Chopped chives or parsley for garnish (optional)

Instructions:

1. In a large skillet, cook the turkey bacon over medium heat until crispy, about 5•7 minutes per side. Transfer the cooked bacon to a paper towel•lined plate.

2. Drain all but 1 tbsp of the bacon grease from the skillet.

3. Crack the eggs directly into the skillet with the remaining bacon grease.

4. Cook the eggs for 2•3 minutes for sunny•side up, or until the whites are set but the yolks are still runny.

5. Alternatively, you can scramble the eggs by gently stirring and folding them in the skillet until cooked through.

6. Season the eggs with salt and pepper to taste.

7. Arrange the cooked turkey bacon slices alongside the eggs on the plates.

8. Garnish with chopped chives or parsley, if desired.

Serve the turkey bacon and eggs immediately, while hot.

The lean turkey bacon provides a nice smoky, savory contrast to the rich, runny eggs. This makes a satisfying and protein•packed breakfast or brunch. Enjoy!

20. Egg muffins with bacon bits

Ingredient:

- 8 large eggs
- 1/4 cup milk
- 1/2 tsp salt
- 1/4 tsp black pepper
- 1/2 cup cooked bacon, crumbled
- 1/2 cup shredded cheddar cheese
- Chopped chives or green onions for garnish (optional)

Instructions:

1. Preheat your oven to 350°F (175°C). Grease a 12•cup muffin tin.

2. In a medium bowl, whisk together the eggs, milk, salt, and pepper until well combined.

3. Divide the crumbled bacon evenly among the muffin cups.

4. Carefully pour the egg mixture over the bacon, filling each cup about 3/4 full.

5. Sprinkle the shredded cheddar cheese over the top of the egg mixture in each cup.

6. Bake for 18•22 minutes, or until the eggs are set and the tops are lightly golden.

7. Remove the egg muffins from the oven and let them cool in the tin for 5 minutes.

8. Use a butter knife or small spatula to gently remove the egg muffins from the tin.

9. Serve the egg muffins warm, garnished with chopped chives or green onions if desired.

These portable egg muffins are perfect for a quick breakfast or snack. The bacon and cheese add delicious savory flavors. They can also be made ahead of time and reheated as needed. Enjoy!

21. Carnivore frittata

Ingredient:

- 8 eggs
- 1/4 cup heavy cream
- 1/2 tsp salt
- 1/4 tsp black pepper
- 1 tbsp olive oil
- 1/2 lb ground breakfast sausage, cooked and crumbled
- 1/2 lb bacon, cooked and crumbled
- 1/2 cup diced ham or prosciutto
- 1 cup shredded cheddar cheese

Instructions:

1. Preheat your oven to 375°F (190°C).

2. In a large bowl, whisk together the eggs, heavy cream, salt, and pepper until well combined.

3. Heat the olive oil in a 10•inch oven•safe skillet over medium heat.

4. Add the cooked and crumbled sausage, bacon, and diced ham/prosciutto to the skillet. Stir to distribute evenly.

5. Pour the egg mixture over the meat in the skillet. Sprinkle the shredded cheddar cheese on top.

6. Transfer the skillet to the preheated oven and bake for 18•22 minutes, or until the center of the frittata is set.

7. Remove the frittata from the oven and let it cool for 5 minutes.

8. Slice the frittata and serve warm.

This carnivore•friendly frittata is packed with savory meats like sausage, bacon, and ham. The eggs and cheese create a rich, satisfying dish that's perfect for breakfast, brunch, or even a light dinner. Enjoy!

22. Venison sausage and eggs

Ingredient:

- 8 oz venison sausage, casings removed
- 1 tbsp olive oil
- 6 large eggs
- 2 tbsp milk
- 2 tbsp chopped fresh parsley
- Salt and pepper to taste

Instructions:

1. In a large skillet, cook the venison sausage over medium•high heat, breaking it up with a spatula as it cooks, until browned and cooked through, about 5•7 minutes. Transfer the cooked sausage to a plate and set aside.

2. In the same skillet, heat the olive oil over medium heat.

3. In a medium bowl, whisk together the eggs and milk until well combined. Season with salt and pepper.

4. Pour the egg mixture into the hot skillet. Use a spatula to gently push the eggs from the edges of the pan towards the center, tilting the pan to allow the uncooked egg to flow to the edges. Continue doing this until the eggs are softly scrambled, about 2•3 minutes.

5. Remove the skillet from the heat and stir in the cooked venison sausage and chopped parsley.

6. Serve the venison sausage and scrambled eggs immediately, while hot.

The lean, flavorful venison sausage pairs perfectly with the fluffy scrambled eggs. This makes a hearty and protein•packed breakfast or brunch dish. Enjoy!

23. Canadian bacon and eggs

Ingredient:

- 4 slices Canadian bacon
- 4 large eggs
- 1 tbsp butter
- Salt and pepper to taste
- Chopped chives or parsley for garnish (optional)

Instructions:

1. In a large skillet, cook the Canadian bacon over medium heat for 2•3 minutes per side, until lightly browned. Transfer the cooked bacon to a plate and set aside.

2. In the same skillet, melt the butter over medium heat.

3. Crack the eggs directly into the skillet. Cook for 2•3 minutes for sunny•side up, or until the whites are set but the yolks are still runny.

4. Alternatively, you can scramble the eggs by gently stirring and folding them in the skillet until cooked through.

5. Season the eggs with salt and pepper to taste.

6. Arrange the cooked Canadian bacon slices alongside the eggs on the plates.

7. Garnish with chopped chives or parsley, if desired.

Serve the Canadian bacon and eggs immediately, while hot.

The savory, slightly salty Canadian bacon pairs perfectly with the rich, runny eggs. This makes a classic and satisfying breakfast or brunch dish. Enjoy!

24. Chorizo and eggs

Ingredient:

- 8 oz Mexican chorizo sausage, casings removed
- 1 tbsp olive oil
- 6 large eggs
- 2 tbsp milk
- 2 tbsp chopped cilantro
- Salt and pepper to taste

Instructions:

1. In a large skillet, cook the chorizo over medium•high heat, breaking it up with a spatula as it cooks, until browned and cooked through, about 5•7 minutes. Transfer the cooked chorizo to a plate and set aside.

2. In the same skillet, heat the olive oil over medium heat.

3. In a medium bowl, whisk together the eggs and milk until well combined. Season with salt and pepper.

4. Pour the egg mixture into the hot skillet. Use a spatula to gently push the eggs from the edges of the pan towards the center, tilting the pan to allow the uncooked egg to flow to the edges. Continue doing this until the eggs are softly scrambled, about 2•3 minutes.

5. Remove the skillet from the heat and stir in the cooked chorizo and chopped cilantro.

6. Serve the chorizo and scrambled eggs immediately, while hot.

The spicy, flavorful chorizo sausage adds a delicious kick to the fluffy scrambled eggs. This makes a hearty and protein•packed breakfast or brunch dish. Enjoy!

25. Breakfast steak with mushrooms

Ingredient:

- 2 (6•8 oz) beef tenderloin steaks, about 1•inch thick
- 2 tbsp olive oil
- 8 oz sliced mushrooms
- 2 cloves garlic, minced
- 2 tbsp unsalted butter
- 2 tbsp heavy cream
- Salt and pepper to taste
- Chopped parsley for garnish (optional)

Instructions:

1. Season the steaks generously with salt and pepper on both sides.

2. Heat 1 tbsp of the olive oil in a large skillet over medium•high heat. Add the steaks and cook for 3•4 minutes per side for medium•rare, or until they reach your desired doneness. Transfer the cooked steaks to a plate and let them rest.

3. In the same skillet, heat the remaining 1 tbsp of olive oil over medium•high heat. Add the sliced mushrooms and cook for 5•7 minutes, stirring occasionally, until the mushrooms are browned and tender.

4. Add the minced garlic to the skillet and cook for 1 minute, until fragrant.

5. Reduce the heat to low and stir in the butter and heavy cream. Cook for 2•3 minutes, stirring frequently, until the sauce thickens slightly.

6. Slice the rested steaks and arrange them on plates. Top with the creamy mushroom sauce.

7. Garnish with chopped parsley if desired.

Serve the breakfast steak with mushrooms immediately, while hot. This makes a decadent and satisfying breakfast or brunch dish. Enjoy!

26. Grilled chicken breast

Ingredient:

- 4 boneless, skinless chicken breasts
- 2 tbsp olive oil
- 1 tsp garlic powder
- 1 tsp onion powder
- 1 tsp dried oregano
- 1 tsp paprika
- Salt and pepper to taste

Instructions:

1. Preheat your grill or grill pan to medium•high heat.

2. Pat the chicken breasts dry with paper towels and place them in a shallow dish or resealable bag.

3. In a small bowl, mix together the olive oil, garlic powder, onion powder, oregano, paprika, salt, and pepper.

4. Pour the seasoning mixture over the chicken breasts and rub it in evenly to coat all sides.

5. Grill the chicken for 5•7 minutes per side, or until the internal temperature reaches 165°F (75°C) when measured with a meat thermometer.

6. Transfer the grilled chicken breasts to a clean cutting board and let them rest for 5 minutes before slicing or serving.

Tips:
- Pound the chicken breasts to an even thickness before grilling for more even cooking.
- Baste the chicken with any remaining seasoning mixture during the last few minutes of grilling.
- Serve the grilled chicken breasts whole or slice them and add to salads, wraps, or other dishes.

This simple grilled chicken breast recipe is a great protein•packed option for a healthy meal. Enjoy!

27. Ribeye steak

Ingredient:

- 2 (8•10 oz) ribeye steaks, about 1•inch thick
- 2 tbsp olive oil
- 2 tsp coarse sea salt
- 1 tsp freshly ground black pepper

Instructions:

1. Remove the steaks from the refrigerator and let them come to room temperature, about 30 minutes.

2. Pat the steaks dry with paper towels and generously season both sides with the salt and pepper.

3. Heat a cast•iron skillet or heavy•duty grill pan over high heat. Add the olive oil and swirl to coat the bottom of the pan.

4. When the pan is very hot, add the ribeye steaks. Cook for 4•5 minutes per side for medium•rare, or longer if you prefer a different doneness.

5. Use tongs to sear the edges of the steaks as well, about 1 minute per side.

6. Transfer the cooked steaks to a cutting board and let them rest for 5•10 minutes before slicing.

7. Slice the ribeye steaks against the grain and serve immediately.

Tips:
- Use an instant•read thermometer to check the internal temperature. Medium•rare is 130•135°F, medium is 140•145°F.
- Baste the steaks with the hot pan juices while cooking for extra flavor.
- Serve the ribeye steaks with your choice of sides, such as roasted vegetables or a fresh salad.

This simple preparation allows the natural flavor of the high•quality ribeye steak to shine. Enjoy this juicy, tender, and flavorful cut of meat!

28. Beef burger patties (no bun)

Ingredient:

- 1 lb ground beef
- 1 tsp salt
- 1/2 tsp black pepper
- 1/2 tsp garlic powder
- 1/2 tsp onion powder
- 1 tbsp Worcestershire sauce (optional)
- Toppings of your choice (e.g. cheese, lettuce, tomato, onion)

Instructions:

1. In a large bowl, gently mix together the ground beef, salt, black pepper, garlic powder, onion powder, and Worcestershire sauce (if using) until just combined. Be careful not to overmix.

2. Divide the beef mixture into 4-6 equal portions and shape them into patties, each about 1/2 inch thick.

3. Preheat your grill, grill pan, or cast-iron skillet over medium-high heat.

4. Cook the burger patties for 4-5 minutes per side, or until they reach your desired level of doneness. Use a meat thermometer to ensure they reach an internal temperature of 160°F (71°C) for medium.

5. Transfer the cooked burger patties to a plate and let them rest for 5 minutes.

6. Serve the beef burger patties with your desired toppings, such as cheese, lettuce, tomato, and onion. You can also serve them with a side salad or roasted vegetables for a low-carb meal.

These bun-less beef burger patties are a great option for those following a keto or low-carb diet. The simple seasoning allows the flavor of the beef to shine. Enjoy!

29. Pork ribs

Ingredient:

- 2 racks of pork baby back ribs (about 3•4 lbs total)
- 2 tbsp brown sugar
- 2 tsp smoked paprika
- 1 tsp garlic powder
- 1 tsp onion powder
- 1 tsp salt
- 1/2 tsp black pepper
- 1 cup barbecue sauce (your favorite)

Instructions:

1. Preheat your oven to 300°F (150°C).

2. Remove the thin membrane from the back of the ribs by sliding a butter knife under it and gently peeling it off. This will help the seasoning and sauce penetrate the meat better.

3. In a small bowl, mix together the brown sugar, smoked paprika, garlic powder, onion powder, salt, and black pepper.

4. Rub the seasoning mixture all over both sides of the ribs, pressing it in to adhere.

5. Place the seasoned ribs in a large baking dish or on a rimmed baking sheet. Cover tightly with aluminum foil.

6. Bake the ribs for 2•2.5 hours, or until the meat is very tender and starting to pull away from the bones.

7. Remove the ribs from the oven and brush them generously with the barbecue sauce, coating both sides.

8. Return the ribs to the oven, uncovered, and bake for an additional 15•20 minutes to caramelize the sauce.

9. Let the ribs rest for 5•10 minutes before slicing and serving.

Serve the pork ribs hot, with any extra barbecue sauce on the side for dipping. Enjoy these tender, flavorful ribs!

30. Lamb kebabs

Ingredient:

- 1 lb lamb, cut into 1·inch cubes
- 1 red onion, cut into 1·inch pieces
- 1 red bell pepper, cut into 1·inch pieces
- 8 oz mushrooms, halved
- 2 tbsp olive oil
- 2 tsp dried oregano
- 1 tsp ground cumin
- 1 tsp paprika
- 1/2 tsp salt
- 1/4 tsp black pepper
- Lemon wedges for serving

Instructions:

1. In a large bowl, combine the lamb cubes, onion, bell pepper, and mushrooms.

2. In a small bowl, whisk together the olive oil, oregano, cumin, paprika, salt, and black pepper.

3. Pour the seasoning mixture over the lamb and vegetables and toss to coat everything evenly.

4. Thread the marinated lamb and vegetables onto metal or wooden skewers, alternating the ingredients.

5. Preheat your grill or grill pan to medium·high heat.

6. Grill the lamb kebabs for 8·10 minutes, turning occasionally, until the lamb is cooked through and the vegetables are tender. Serve the grilled lamb kebabs immediately, with lemon wedges on the side.

Tips:
- Soak wooden skewers in water for 30 minutes before using to prevent them from burning.
- Adjust the cooking time based on the thickness of your lamb cubes and desired doneness.
- You can also broil the lamb kebabs in the oven for 10·12 minutes, turning halfway through.

31. Baked salmon fillet

Ingredient:

- 1 lb salmon fillet, skin•on or skin•off
- 2 tbsp olive oil
- 1 tsp lemon zest
- 2 tbsp lemon juice
- 2 cloves garlic, minced
- 1 tsp dried dill
- 1/2 tsp salt
- 1/4 tsp black pepper

Instructions:

1. Preheat your oven to 400°F (200°C).

2. Place the salmon fillet in a baking dish or on a rimmed baking sheet lined with parchment paper.

3. In a small bowl, whisk together the olive oil, lemon zest, lemon juice, garlic, dried dill, salt, and black pepper.

4. Pour the lemon•garlic mixture over the salmon, making sure to coat the top and sides of the fillet.

5. Bake the salmon for 12•15 minutes, or until it flakes easily with a fork and reaches an internal temperature of 145°F (63°C).

6. Remove the baked salmon from the oven and let it rest for 5 minutes.

7. Serve the salmon fillet warm, garnished with additional lemon wedges if desired.

Tips:
- For a crispy skin, broil the salmon for the last 2•3 minutes of cooking.
- Adjust the baking time based on the thickness of your salmon fillet.
- Pair the baked salmon with roasted vegetables, a fresh salad, or steamed rice for a complete meal.

This simple baked salmon recipe results in a tender, flavorful fillet that's perfect for a healthy and delicious dinner. Enjoy!

32. Grilled shrimp skewers

Ingredient:

- 1 lb large shrimp, peeled and deveined
- 2 tbsp olive oil
- 2 tbsp lemon juice
- 2 cloves garlic, minced
- 1 tsp dried oregano
- 1/2 tsp paprika
- 1/4 tsp red pepper flakes (optional)
- Salt and pepper to taste
- Wooden or metal skewers

Instructions:

1. If using wooden skewers, soak them in water for 30 minutes to prevent them from burning on the grill.

2. In a large bowl, combine the shrimp, olive oil, lemon juice, garlic, oregano, paprika, red pepper flakes (if using), salt, and pepper. Toss to coat the shrimp evenly.

3. Thread the marinated shrimp onto the skewers, leaving a little space between each one.

4. Preheat your grill or grill pan to medium•high heat.

5. Grill the shrimp skewers for 2•3 minutes per side, or until the shrimp are opaque and cooked through.

6. Transfer the grilled shrimp skewers to a serving platter.

7. Serve the shrimp skewers immediately, garnished with lemon wedges if desired.

Tips:
- Soak wooden skewers in water to prevent them from burning on the grill.
- Adjust the amount of red pepper flakes to control the level of spiciness.
- Grill the shrimp skewers in batches if necessary to avoid overcrowding the grill.

These flavorful grilled shrimp skewers make a delicious and easy•to•prepare appetizer or main dish. Enjoy!

33. Meatza (pizza with a meat crust)

Ingredient:

- 1 lb ground beef
- 1 lb Italian sausage, casings removed
- 1 egg
- 1/2 cup grated Parmesan cheese
- 1 tsp dried oregano
- 1/2 tsp garlic powder
- 1/2 tsp onion powder
- 1/4 tsp red pepper flakes (optional)
- Salt and pepper to taste
- Desired pizza toppings (e.g. tomato sauce, cheese, vegetables)

Instructions:

1. Preheat your oven to 400°F (200°C). Line a large baking sheet or pizza pan with parchment paper.

2. In a large bowl, combine the ground beef, Italian sausage, egg, Parmesan cheese, oregano, garlic powder, onion powder, red pepper flakes (if using), salt, and pepper. Mix until well incorporated.

3. Press the meat mixture evenly into the prepared baking sheet or pizza pan, forming a thin, even crust.

4. Bake the meat crust for 15•20 minutes, or until it's cooked through and starting to brown on the edges.

5. Remove the partially baked crust from the oven and top it with your desired pizza toppings, such as tomato sauce, shredded cheese, and vegetables.

6. Return the topped meatza to the oven and bake for an additional 10•15 minutes, or until the cheese is melted and bubbly.

7. Slice and serve the meatza hot.

Tips:
- Use a combination of ground beef and Italian sausage for the best flavor.
- Adjust the baking time as needed, depending on the thickness of your meat crust.
- For a crispier crust, you can broil the meatza for the last 2•3 minutes of cooking.

34. Chicken drumsticks

Ingredient:

- 8 chicken drumsticks
- 2 tbsp olive oil
- 1 tsp paprika
- 1 tsp garlic powder
- 1 tsp onion powder
- 1 tsp dried thyme
- 1 tsp salt
- 1/2 tsp black pepper

Instructions:

1. Preheat your oven to 400°F (200°C). Line a large baking sheet with parchment paper or foil.

2. Pat the chicken drumsticks dry with paper towels and place them in a large bowl.

3. In a small bowl, mix together the olive oil, paprika, garlic powder, onion powder, dried thyme, salt, and black pepper.

4. Pour the seasoning mixture over the chicken drumsticks and toss to coat them evenly.

5. Arrange the seasoned drumsticks in a single layer on the prepared baking sheet.

6. Bake the chicken for 35·40 minutes, flipping the drumsticks halfway through, until the skin is crispy and the internal temperature reaches 165°F (75°C).

7. Remove the baked chicken drumsticks from the oven and let them rest for 5 minutes.

8. Serve the chicken drumsticks hot, garnished with chopped parsley if desired.

Tips:
- For extra crispy skin, broil the drumsticks for the last 2·3 minutes of cooking.
- Adjust the baking time baood on the size of your drumsticks
- Serve the baked chicken drumsticks with your favorite sides, such as roasted vegetables or a fresh salad.

35. T•bone steak

Ingredient:

- 1 (1.5•2 lb) T•bone steak, about 1•inch thick
- 2 tbsp olive oil
- 2 tsp coarse sea salt
- 1 tsp freshly ground black pepper

Instructions:

1. Remove the T•bone steak from the refrigerator and let it come to room temperature, about 30 minutes.

2. Pat the steak dry with paper towels and generously season both sides with the salt and pepper.

3. Preheat your grill or grill pan to high heat.

4. Brush the steak lightly with the olive oil on both sides.

5. Grill the T•bone steak for 4•6 minutes per side, depending on thickness, for medium•rare doneness. Use tongs to sear the edges as well.

6. Use an instant•read thermometer to check the internal temperature. For medium•rare, aim for 130•135°F. For medium, 140•145°F.

7. Transfer the grilled T•bone steak to a cutting board and let it rest for 5•10 minutes.

8. Slice the steak across the grain and serve immediately.

Tips:
- Let the steak come to room temperature before grilling for more even cooking.
- Use the "flip frequently" method, flipping the steak every 1•2 minutes, for a nice crust.
- Baste the steak with any accumulated juices while resting for extra flavor.
- Serve the T•bone steak with your choice of sides, such as roasted potatoes or a fresh salad.

The T•bone steak is a flavorful and tender cut that's perfect for grilling. Enjoy this juicy, perfectly cooked steak!

36. Roast beef slices

Ingredient:

- 2 lbs beef roast (such as top round, eye of round, or chuck roast)
- 2 tbsp olive oil
- 2 tsp salt
- 1 tsp black pepper
- 1 tsp garlic powder
- 1 tsp onion powder

Instructions:

1. Preheat your oven to 450°F (230°C).

2. Pat the beef roast dry with paper towels and place it in a roasting pan or on a rimmed baking sheet.

3. In a small bowl, mix together the olive oil, salt, black pepper, garlic powder, and onion powder.

4. Rub the seasoning mixture all over the surface of the beef roast, making sure to coat it evenly.

5. Roast the beef for 15 minutes, then reduce the oven temperature to 300°F (150°C) and continue roasting for 1•1.5 hours, or until the internal temperature reaches 125•130°F (52•54°C) for medium•rare.

6. Remove the roast from the oven and let it rest for 15•20 minutes before slicing.

7. Using a sharp knife, slice the roast beef across the grain into thin, even slices.

8. Serve the roast beef slices warm, or refrigerate and serve chilled.

Tips:
- Use a meat thermometer to ensure the roast reaches your desired level of doneness.
- For a more well•done roast, cook it to an internal temperature of 135•140°F (57•60°C).
- Slice the roast beef against the grain for the most tender slices.
- Serve the roast beef slices with your favorite condiments, such as horseradish, mustard, or au jus.

37. Pork chops

Ingredient:

• 4 bone•in pork chops, about 1•inch thick
• 2 tbsp olive oil
• 1 tsp garlic powder
• 1 tsp onion powder
• 1 tsp dried thyme
• 1 tsp salt
• 1/2 tsp black pepper

Instructions:

1. Preheat your oven to 400°F (200°C). Lightly grease a baking dish or line a baking sheet with parchment paper.

2. Pat the pork chops dry with paper towels and place them in a large bowl.

3. In a small bowl, mix together the olive oil, garlic powder, onion powder, dried thyme, salt, and black pepper.

4. Pour the seasoning mixture over the pork chops and use your hands to rub it in, making sure to coat both sides evenly.

5. Arrange the seasoned pork chops in a single layer in the prepared baking dish or on the baking sheet.

6. Bake the pork chops for 18•22 minutes, flipping them halfway through, until they reach an internal temperature of 145°F (63°C).

7. Remove the baked pork chops from the oven and let them rest for 5 minutes before serving.

Tips:
• Adjust the baking time based on the thickness of your pork chops.
• For extra crispy edges, broil the pork chops for the last 2•3 minutes of cooking.
• Serve the baked pork chops with your choice of sides, such as roasted vegetables or a fresh salad.

These simple, flavorful baked pork chops make a delicious and easy•to•prepare main dish. Enjoy!

38. Lamb shank

Ingredient:

- 4 lamb shanks
- 2 tbsp olive oil
- 1 onion, diced
- 3 carrots, peeled and diced
- 3 celery stalks, diced
- 4 garlic cloves, minced
- 1 cup red wine
- 2 cups beef or chicken broth
- 1 (14.5 oz) can diced tomatoes
- 2 bay leaves
- 2 sprigs fresh thyme
- 1 tsp dried rosemary
- Salt and pepper to taste

Instructions:

1. Preheat your oven to 325°F (165°C).

2. Season the lamb shanks generously with salt and pepper.

3. In a large, oven•safe Dutch oven or heavy•bottomed pot, heat the olive oil over medium•high heat. Sear the lamb shanks on all sides until browned, about 3•4 minutes per side. Transfer the shanks to a plate.

4. Reduce the heat to medium and add the onion, carrots, celery, and garlic to the pot. Cook for 5•7 minutes, stirring occasionally, until the vegetables are softened.

5. Pour in the red wine and use a wooden spoon to scrape up any browned bits from the bottom of the pot.

6. Add the broth, diced tomatoes, bay leaves, thyme, and rosemary. Bring the mixture to a simmer.

7. Return the seared lamb shanks to the pot, cover, and transfer to the preheated oven.

8. Braise the lamb shanks for 2•2.5 hours, or until the meat is very tender and falling off the bone.

9. Remove the pot from the oven and let the lamb shanks rest for 10 minutes.

10. Serve the braised lamb shanks warm, with the cooking liquid spooned over the top. Enjoy!

39. Duck breast

Ingredient:

- 2 duck breasts, skin•on
- 1 tsp salt
- 1/2 tsp black pepper
- 1 tbsp olive oil

Instructions:

1. Pat the duck breasts dry with paper towels and use a sharp knife to score the skin in a crosshatch pattern, being careful not to cut into the meat.

2. Season the duck breasts all over with the salt and pepper.

3. Heat a large, oven•safe skillet over medium•high heat. Add the olive oil.

4. Place the duck breasts skin•side down in the hot skillet. Cook for 5•7 minutes, or until the skin is crispy and golden brown.

5. Flip the duck breasts over and transfer the skillet to a preheated 400°F (200°C) oven.

6. Roast the duck for an additional 8•10 minutes for medium•rare, or 10•12 minutes for medium doneness.

7. Remove the skillet from the oven and transfer the duck breasts to a cutting board. Let them rest for 5•10 minutes.

8. Slice the duck breasts against the grain and serve immediately.

Tips:
- Use a meat thermometer to ensure the duck reaches your desired doneness. Medium•rare is 130°F, medium is 140°F.
- Render the fat from the skin by scoring it before cooking.
- Serve the seared duck breast with roasted vegetables, a fresh salad, or a fruit compote.

The crispy skin and juicy, tender meat of the duck breast make this an impressive and delicious meal. Enjoy!

40. Beef stew (meat only)

Ingredient:

- 2 lbs beef chuck, cut into 1•inch cubes
- 2 tbsp olive oil
- 1 onion, diced
- 3 cloves garlic, minced
- 2 cups beef broth
- 1 cup dry red wine
- 2 bay leaves
- 2 sprigs fresh thyme
- 1 tsp dried oregano
- 1 tsp paprika
- Salt and pepper to taste

Instructions:

1. In a large Dutch oven or heavy•bottomed pot, heat the olive oil over medium•high heat.

2. Working in batches if necessary, sear the beef cubes on all sides until browned, about 2•3 minutes per side. Transfer the seared beef to a plate.

3. Reduce the heat to medium and add the diced onion to the pot. Cook for 5•7 minutes, stirring occasionally, until the onion is softened.

4. Add the minced garlic and cook for 1 minute, until fragrant.

5. Pour in the beef broth and red wine, scraping up any browned bits from the bottom of the pot.

6. Add the bay leaves, thyme sprigs, oregano, and paprika. Season with salt and pepper to taste.

7. Return the seared beef cubes to the pot and bring the mixture to a simmer.

8. Cover the pot, transfer it to the oven, and braise the beef for 2•2.5 hours, or until the meat is very tender.

9. Remove the pot from the oven and discard the bay leaves and thyme sprigs.. Serve the braised beef stew meat as is, or over mashed cauliflower or zucchini noodles for a low•carb meal.

41. Smoked brisket

Ingredient:

- 4•5 lb beef brisket, trimmed of excess fat
- 2 tbsp coarse sea salt
- 2 tbsp black pepper
- 1 tbsp garlic powder
- 1 tbsp onion powder
- 1 tbsp smoked paprika
- Wood chips for smoking (such as oak, hickory, or mesquite)

Instructions:

1. Pat the brisket dry with paper towels and place it on a large cutting board or baking sheet.

2. In a small bowl, mix together the salt, black pepper, garlic powder, onion powder, and smoked paprika. Rub the seasoning mixture all over the brisket, covering all sides.

3. Prepare your smoker according to the manufacturer's instructions. Soak the wood chips in water for 30 minutes before adding them to the smoker.

4. Place the seasoned brisket in the smoker, fat•side up. Smoke the brisket for 6•8 hours, or until it reaches an internal temperature of 195•205°F (91•96°C).

5. Wrap the smoked brisket tightly in foil or butcher paper and let it rest for 1•2 hours.

6. Unwrap the brisket and slice it against the grain into thin, even slices.

7. Serve the smoked brisket warm, with your favorite barbecue sauce, pickles, and sides.

Tips:
- Trim the brisket to remove any excess fat, leaving a 1/4•inch fat cap.
- Maintain a consistent smoker temperature between 225•250°F (107•121°C) for best results.
- Spritz the brisket with apple juice or beef broth every 1•2 hours during smoking to keep it moist.
- Let the brisket rest for at least 1 hour before slicing to allow the juices to redistribute.

42. Roast turkey

Ingredient:

- 12•14 lb whole turkey, thawed if frozen
- 1 cup unsalted butter, softened
- 2 tbsp chopped fresh sage
- 2 tbsp chopped fresh thyme
- 1 tbsp chopped fresh rosemary
- 1 tsp salt
- 1/2 tsp black pepper
- 1 onion, quartered
- 2 carrots, cut into 2•inch pieces
- 2 celery stalks, cut into 2•inch pieces
- 4 cups turkey or chicken broth

Instructions:

1. Preheat your oven to 325°F (165°C).

2. Remove the giblets and neck from the turkey cavity and discard or save for another use. Pat the turkey dry with paper towels.

3. In a small bowl, mix together the softened butter, chopped sage, thyme, rosemary, salt, and pepper.

4. Gently loosen the skin of the turkey and spread half of the herb butter mixture under the skin, covering the breast and legs. Spread the remaining butter mixture over the outside of the turkey.

5. Place the onion, carrots, and celery in the bottom of a large roasting pan. Set the turkey, breast•side up, on top of the vegetables.

6. Pour the broth into the bottom of the roasting pan.

7. Roast the turkey for 2.5•3 hours, basting every 30 minutes with the pan juices, until the internal temperature reaches 165°F (74°C) in the thickest part of the breast and 175°F (79°C) in the thigh.

8. Transfer the roasted turkey to a cutting board and let it rest for 30 minutes before carving and serving.

43. Stuffed pork tenderloin (with cheese)

Ingredient:

- 1 lb pork tenderloin
- 4 oz cream cheese, softened
- 1/2 cup shredded cheddar cheese
- 2 tbsp chopped fresh parsley
- 1 tsp garlic powder
- 1/2 tsp salt
- 1/4 tsp black pepper

Instructions:

1. Preheat your oven to 400°F (200°C).

2. Slice the pork tenderloin lengthwise, being careful not to cut all the way through. Open the tenderloin like a book and pound it lightly with a meat mallet to flatten it into an even thickness.

3. In a small bowl, mix together the cream cheese, cheddar cheese, parsley, garlic powder, salt, and black pepper until well combined.

4. Spread the cheese mixture evenly over the flattened pork tenderloin, leaving a 1·inch border on all sides.

5. Carefully roll up the pork tenderloin, starting from the short end, and secure it with kitchen twine or toothpicks.

6. Place the stuffed pork tenderloin in a baking dish or on a rimmed baking sheet.

7. Roast the stuffed pork tenderloin for 25·30 minutes, or until the internal temperature reaches 145°F (63°C).

8. Remove the pork from the oven and let it rest for 5·10 minutes before slicing and serving.

This cheesy, flavorful stuffed pork tenderloin makes for an impressive and delicious main dish. Enjoy!

44. Bison burger patties

Ingredient:

- 1 lb ground bison meat
- 1 tsp salt
- 1/2 tsp black pepper
- 1 tsp Worcestershire sauce
- 1 tbsp olive oil

Instructions:

1. In a large bowl, gently mix together the ground bison, salt, pepper, and Worcestershire sauce until just combined. Be careful not to overmix.

2. Divide the bison mixture into 4•6 equal portions and gently form them into patties, about 3/4 inch thick. Try not to pack the patties too tightly.

3. Heat the olive oil in a large skillet or grill pan over medium•high heat.

4. Add the bison patties and cook for 4•5 minutes per side, or until they reach your desired doneness. Bison cooks faster than beef, so be careful not to overcook.

5. Transfer the cooked bison burgers to a plate and let them rest for 5 minutes before serving.

Serving Suggestions:

- Serve the bison burgers on toasted buns with your favorite toppings like cheese, lettuce, tomato, onion, etc.

- For a low•carb option, serve the patties on a bed of greens or wrapped in lettuce leaves.

- Top with sautéed mushrooms, caramelized onions, or a dollop of garlic aioli.

Tips:
- Handle the bison meat gently to prevent the patties from becoming tough.
- Bison is a lean meat, so be careful not to overcook it or it can become dry.
- You can also grill the bison patties over medium•high heat for 4•5 minutes per side.

Enjoy your delicious and healthy bison burger patties!

45. Grilled sausages

Ingredient:

- 6-8 Italian sausages or bratwurst
- 1 tbsp olive oil
- Salt and pepper to taste

Instructions:

1. Preheat your grill to medium-high heat.

2. Brush the sausages lightly with olive oil and season with salt and pepper.

3. Place the sausages directly on the grill grates. Grill for 12-15 minutes, turning occasionally, until the sausages are cooked through and have nice grill marks.

4. Transfer the grilled sausages to a serving platter.

5. Serve the grilled sausages hot, with your favorite toppings or sides such as sauerkraut, mustard, rolls, or potato salad.

Tips:
- For extra flavor, you can add some herbs like rosemary or thyme to the olive oil before brushing the sausages.

- Be careful not to overcrowd the grill, cook the sausages in batches if needed.

- Use tongs to turn the sausages, avoid piercing them with a fork which can cause the juices to leak out.

- Let the sausages rest for 5 minutes before serving to allow the juices to redistribute.

46. Veal cutlets

Ingredient:

- 4 veal cutlets, about 1/2 inch thick
- 1/2 cup all•purpose flour
- 2 eggs, beaten
- 1 cup breadcrumbs
- 1/4 cup grated Parmesan cheese
- 1 tsp dried parsley
- 1/2 tsp salt
- 1/4 tsp black pepper
- 2 tbsp olive oil

Instructions:

1. Prepare the breading station. Place the flour in one shallow dish, the beaten eggs in another, and the breadcrumbs mixed with Parmesan, parsley, salt, and pepper in a third dish.

2. Dredge the veal cutlets in the flour, dip them in the beaten egg, and then coat them evenly with the breadcrumb mixture, pressing gently to adhere.

3. Heat the olive oil in a large skillet over medium•high heat.

4. Working in batches if needed, add the breaded veal cutlets to the hot oil and cook for 2•3 minutes per side, until golden brown and cooked through.

5. Transfer the cooked veal cutlets to a paper towel•lined plate to drain any excess oil. Serve the veal cutlets hot, garnished with lemon wedges if desired.

Serving Suggestions:
- Serve the veal cutlets with a side of roasted potatoes, a fresh salad, or steamed vegetables.
- Top the cutlets with a lemon•caper sauce or a creamy mushroom sauce.
- Use the veal cutlets to make veal parmesan or veal Milanese.

Tips:
- Pound the veal cutlets lightly between two sheets of plastic wrap to tenderize them.
- Refrigerate the breaded cutlets for 30 minutes before frying to help the breading adhere better.
- Use high•quality, fresh veal for the best flavor and texture.

47. Bacon•wrapped chicken thighs

Ingredient:

• 8 boneless, skinless chicken thighs
• 8 slices of bacon
• 1 tsp smoked paprika
• 1 tsp garlic powder
• 1/2 tsp salt
• 1/4 tsp black pepper

Instructions:

1. Preheat your oven to 400°F (200°C).

2. In a small bowl, mix together the smoked paprika, garlic powder, salt, and black pepper.

3. Season the chicken thighs all over with the spice mixture.

4. Wrap each chicken thigh tightly with a slice of bacon, securing it with a toothpick if needed.

5. Arrange the bacon•wrapped chicken thighs in a single layer on a baking sheet or in a baking dish.

6. Bake for 35•40 minutes, or until the chicken is cooked through and the bacon is crispy. Remove the toothpicks before serving.

Serving Suggestions:
• Serve the bacon•wrapped chicken thighs with roasted vegetables, mashed potatoes, or a fresh salad.
• For extra flavor, you can brush the chicken with a glaze made from honey, mustard, or barbecue sauce during the last 10 minutes of baking.
• Sprinkle the cooked chicken with chopped fresh parsley or chives for a pop of color and freshness.

Tips:
• Use high•quality, thick•cut bacon for the best results.
• Make sure to wrap the bacon tightly around the chicken to prevent it from unwrapping during baking.
• Adjust the baking time as needed, depending on the size of your chicken thighs.
• Let the chicken rest for 5 minutes before serving to allow the juices to redistribute.

48. Pan•seared scallops

Ingredient:

- 1 lb sea scallops, patted dry with paper towels
- 2 tbsp unsalted butter
- 1 tbsp olive oil
- Salt and pepper to taste
- Lemon wedges for serving (optional)

Instructions:

1. Pat the scallops dry with paper towels and season them with salt and pepper on both sides.

2. Heat a large skillet over high heat. Add the butter and olive oil to the pan.

3. When the butter is melted and the pan is very hot, add the scallops in a single layer, making sure not to overcrowd the pan.

4. Sear the scallops for 2•3 minutes per side, or until they develop a nice golden•brown crust.

5. Avoid moving the scallops too much during the searing process to allow them to develop a good sear.

6. Once the scallops are cooked through and opaque, transfer them to a plate. Serve the pan•seared scallops immediately, with lemon wedges on the side if desired.

Serving Suggestions:
- Serve the scallops over a bed of risotto, pasta, or mixed greens.
- Top the scallops with a drizzle of lemon•garlic butter or a balsamic reduction.
- Pair the scallops with a crisp white wine or a light, refreshing cocktail.

Tips:
- Make sure to pat the scallops very dry before searing to ensure they get a nice, crispy sear.
- Use a high•heat•tolerant oil, like olive oil or avocado oil, to prevent the butter from burning.
- Avoid overcrowding the pan, as this can cause the scallops to steam rather than sear.
- Be careful not to overcook the scallops, as they can become tough and rubbery
- Serve the scallops immediately for the best texture and temperature.

49. Braised short ribs

Ingredient:

- 2 cups red wine
- 2 cups beef broth
- 2 bay leaves
- 2 sprigs fresh thyme
- 1 tsp salt
- 1/2 tsp black pepper

- 3 lbs beef short ribs, cut into 2•inch pieces
- 2 tbsp olive oil
- 1 onion, diced
- 3 carrots, peeled and diced
- 3 celery stalks, diced
- 4 garlic cloves, minced

Instructions:

1. Preheat your oven to 325°F (165°C).

2. Heat the olive oil in a large, oven•safe Dutch oven or heavy•bottomed pot over medium•high heat.

3. Pat the short ribs dry and season them with salt and pepper. Working in batches if needed, sear the short ribs on all sides until they are nicely browned, about 3•4 minutes per side. Transfer the seared ribs to a plate.

4. Reduce the heat to medium and add the onion, carrots, and celery to the pot. Cook, stirring occasionally, until the vegetables are softened, about 5•7 minutes.

5. Add the garlic and cook for an additional minute, until fragrant.

6. Pour in the red wine and use a wooden spoon to scrape up any browned bits from the bottom of the pot.

7. Add the beef broth, bay leaves, and thyme. Bring the mixture to a simmer.

8. Return the seared short ribs to the pot, cover, and transfer to the preheated oven.

9. Braise the short ribs in the oven for 2•3 hours, or until the meat is very tender and falling off the bone.

10. Remove the pot from the oven and transfer the short ribs to a serving platter. Discard the bay leaves and thyme sprigs.. Serve the braised short ribs hot, with the cooking liquid spooned over the top.

50. Corned beef

Ingredient:

- 3·4 lbs corned beef brisket, with seasoning packet
- 1 onion, quartered
- 3 carrots, peeled and cut into 2·inch pieces
- 3 celery stalks, cut into 2·inch pieces
- 4 cloves garlic, peeled
- 1 bay leaf
- 1 tsp whole black peppercorns
- Water or beef broth, enough to cover the brisket

Instructions:

1. Place the corned beef brisket, fat side up, in a large pot or Dutch oven. Add the onion, carrots, celery, garlic, bay leaf, and peppercorns.

2. Pour in enough water or beef broth to just cover the brisket.

3. Bring the liquid to a boil over high heat, then reduce the heat to low, cover the pot, and simmer for 2·3 hours, or until the brisket is very tender.

4. Carefully remove the brisket from the pot and transfer it to a cutting board. Let it rest for 10·15 minutes.

5. Meanwhile, strain the cooking liquid through a fine·mesh sieve, discarding the vegetables and seasonings.

6. Slice the corned beef against the grain into thin slices.

7. Serve the corned beef warm, with the reserved cooking liquid spooned over the top.

Serving Suggestions:
- Serve the corned beef with boiled potatoes, cabbage, and Irish soda bread for a traditional St. Patrick's Day meal.
- Use the corned beef in Reuben sandwiches, hash, or as a topping for shepherd's pie.
- Enjoy the corned beef with a side of mustard, horseradish, or sauerkraut.

Enjoy your delicious homemade corned beef!

51. Fried catfish

Ingredient:

- 1 lb catfish fillets, cut into 4-6 inch pieces
- 1 cup all-purpose flour
- 1 tsp salt
- 1/2 tsp black pepper
- 1/2 tsp paprika
- 1/4 tsp cayenne pepper (optional)
- Vegetable or canola oil for frying

Instructions:

1. Pat the catfish fillets dry with paper towels and set them aside.

2. In a shallow bowl, mix together the flour, salt, black pepper, paprika, and cayenne pepper (if using).

3. Pour enough oil into a large skillet or Dutch oven to reach a depth of about 1/2 inch. Heat the oil over medium-high heat to 350°F (175°C).

4. Working in batches, dredge the catfish fillets in the seasoned flour, coating them evenly on both sides.

5. Carefully add the floured catfish fillets to the hot oil and fry for 3-4 minutes per side, or until they are golden brown and cooked through.

6. Use a slotted spoon or tongs to transfer the fried catfish to a paper towel-lined plate to drain any excess oil.

7. Serve the fried catfish hot, garnished with lemon wedges, if desired.

Serving Suggestions:
- Serve the fried catfish with hush puppies, coleslaw, and tartar sauce.
- Use the fried catfish in a po' boy sandwich with lettuce, tomato, and remoulade sauce.
- Pair the fried catfish with a side of roasted or grilled vegetables.

Enjoy your delicious homemade fried catfish!

52. Venison steak

Ingredient:

- 4 venison steaks, about 1•inch thick
- 2 tbsp olive oil
- 2 tsp salt
- 1 tsp black pepper
- 1 tsp garlic powder
- 1 tsp dried thyme

Instructions:

1. Pat the venison steaks dry with paper towels and let them come to room temperature, about 30 minutes.

2. In a small bowl, mix together the salt, black pepper, garlic powder, and dried thyme.

3. Brush the venison steaks with the olive oil and generously season them on both sides with the spice mixture.

4. Preheat your grill or grill pan to high heat.

5. Grill the venison steaks for 3•5 minutes per side, depending on the thickness, for medium•rare doneness. Adjust the cooking time as needed for your desired level of doneness.

6. Transfer the grilled venison steaks to a cutting board and let them rest for 5•10 minutes before slicing.

7. Slice the venison steaks against the grain and serve immediately.

Serving Suggestions:
- Serve the grilled venison steaks with roasted potatoes, a fresh salad, or sautéed mushrooms and onions.
- Top the venison with a dollop of compound butter, such as garlic•herb or blue cheese butter.
- Pair the venison with a bold red wine, such as a Cabernet Sauvignon or Malbec.

Enjoy your delicious grilled venison steak!

53. Chicken wings

Ingredient:

- 2 lbs chicken wings, drumettes and flats separated
- 2 tbsp baking powder
- 1 tsp salt
- 1/2 tsp black pepper

For the Sauce (optional):
- 1/2 cup hot sauce (such as Frank's RedHot)
- 2 tbsp unsalted butter, melted

Instructions:

1. Preheat your oven to 400°F (200°C). Line a large baking sheet with parchment paper.

2. Pat the chicken wings dry with paper towels. In a large bowl, toss the wings with the baking powder, salt, and pepper until evenly coated.

3. Arrange the wings in a single layer on the prepared baking sheet, making sure they are not touching each other.

4. Bake for 40·45 minutes, flipping the wings halfway through, until they are crispy and golden brown.

5. While the wings are baking, prepare the sauce (if using). In a small bowl, whisk together the hot sauce and melted butter.

6. Once the wings are done, transfer them to a large bowl. If using the sauce, pour it over the wings and toss to coat.

7. Serve the crispy baked chicken wings immediately, with any desired dipping sauces or toppings.

Serving Suggestions:
- Serve the wings with celery sticks, carrot sticks, and blue cheese or ranch dressing.
- Toss the wings in different sauce flavors, such as barbecue, honey garlic, or lemon pepper.
- Sprinkle the wings with chopped fresh parsley or green onions for added flavor and color.

54. Crab legs with butter

Ingredient:

- 2 lbs fresh or frozen crab legs (such as Alaskan king crab or snow crab)
- 1/2 cup unsalted butter, melted
- 2 tbsp fresh lemon juice
- 1 tsp lemon zest
- 1/4 tsp salt
- 1/8 tsp black pepper

Instructions:

1. If using frozen crab legs, thaw them according to the package instructions.

2. Fill a large pot with about 1 inch of water and bring it to a boil over high heat. Place a steamer basket or colander in the pot, making sure the water doesn't touch the bottom.

3. Add the crab legs to the steamer basket, cover the pot with a lid, and steam the crab legs for 5-7 minutes, or until they are heated through and the meat is opaque.

4. While the crab legs are steaming, prepare the lemon butter sauce. In a small bowl, whisk together the melted butter, lemon juice, lemon zest, salt, and black pepper.

5. Carefully transfer the steamed crab legs to a serving platter. Serve the crab legs immediately, with the lemon butter sauce on the side for dipping.

Serving Suggestions:
- Provide small dishes or ramekins for the lemon butter sauce.
- Serve the crab legs with lemon wedges, crusty bread, and a fresh salad or coleslaw.
- For a more indulgent presentation, serve the crab legs on a bed of shredded lettuce or with a side of drawn butter.

Tips:
- Be careful when handling the hot crab legs, as they can be quite delicate.
- Use kitchen shears or a crab cracker to easily break open the crab legs and access the meat.
- Adjust the steaming time as needed, depending on the size and thickness of your crab legs.
- Serve the crab legs immediately for the best texture and temperature.

55. Pan•fried trout

Ingredient:

- 4 trout fillets, about 6•8 oz each
- 1/4 cup all•purpose flour
- 1 tsp salt
- 1/2 tsp black pepper
- 2 tbsp unsalted butter
- 1 tbsp olive oil
- Lemon wedges for serving

Instructions:

1. Pat the trout fillets dry with paper towels and season them on both sides with the salt and pepper.

2. Place the flour in a shallow dish. Dredge the trout fillets in the flour, shaking off any excess.

3. Heat the butter and olive oil in a large skillet over medium•high heat.

4. When the butter is melted and the oil is shimmering, carefully add the floured trout fillets to the pan.

5. Cook the trout for 3•4 minutes per side, or until the fillets are golden brown and cooked through.

6. Transfer the pan•fried trout fillets to a plate and serve immediately, with lemon wedges on the side.

Serving Suggestions:
- Serve the pan•fried trout with a side of roasted vegetables, a fresh salad, or steamed rice.
- Top the trout with a dollop of lemon•herb butter or a drizzle of balsamic reduction.
- Pair the trout with a crisp white wine or a light, citrusy cocktail.

Tips:
- Use fresh, high•quality trout fillets for the best flavor and texture.
- Make sure the oil is hot enough before adding the trout to ensure a crispy, golden•brown crust.
- Avoid overcrowding the pan, as this can cause the trout to steam rather than fry.
- Be careful not to overcook the trout, as it can become dry and tough.
- Serve the pan•fried trout immediately for the best texture and temperature.

56. Filet mignon

Ingredient:

- 4 filet mignon steaks, about 6•8 oz each
- 2 tbsp olive oil
- 2 tsp salt
- 1 tsp black pepper
- 2 tbsp unsalted butter (optional)

Instructions:

1. Remove the filet mignon steaks from the refrigerator and let them come to room temperature, about 30 minutes.

2. Preheat your grill or grill pan to high heat.

3. Pat the filet mignon steaks dry with paper towels and brush them all over with the olive oil. Season them generously with the salt and pepper.

4. Place the seasoned filet mignon steaks on the hot grill and cook for 4•6 minutes per side, depending on the thickness of the steaks, for medium•rare doneness.

5. Use tongs to sear the edges of the steaks, about 1 minute per side, to ensure even cooking.

6. Transfer the grilled filet mignon steaks to a cutting board and let them rest for 5•10 minutes.

7. If desired, top the rested steaks with a pat of unsalted butter and let it melt over the hot meat.

8. Slice the filet mignon steaks and serve immediately.

Serving Suggestions:
- Serve the grilled filet mignon with roasted potatoes, a fresh salad, or sautéed mushrooms and onions.
- Top the steaks with a dollop of compound butter, such as garlic•herb or blue cheese buttor.
- Pair the filet mignon with a full•bodied red wine, such as a Cabernet Sauvignon or Malbec.

57. Prime rib roast

Ingredient:

- 1 (4•5 lb) prime rib roast, bone•in or boneless
- 2 tbsp olive oil
- 2 tbsp coarse salt
- 1 tbsp black pepper
- 2 tbsp chopped fresh rosemary
- 2 tbsp chopped fresh thyme
- 4 cloves garlic, minced

Instructions:

1. Remove the prime rib roast from the refrigerator and let it come to room temperature, about 1 hour.

2. Preheat your oven to 500°F (260°C).

3. In a small bowl, mix together the olive oil, salt, pepper, rosemary, thyme, and garlic to create a paste.

4. Pat the prime rib roast dry with paper towels and generously rub the herb•salt paste all over the surface of the meat, including the sides and ends.

5. Place the seasoned prime rib roast, fat side up, on a wire rack set in a large roasting pan.

6. Roast the prime rib for 15 minutes at 500°F (260°C) to sear the outside.

7. Reduce the oven temperature to 250°F (120°C) and continue roasting the prime rib for 2•3 hours, or until it reaches your desired level of doneness (125°F/52°C for medium•rare, 130°F/54°C for medium).

8. Remove the prime rib roast from the oven and let it rest for 15•20 minutes before slicing. Slice the prime rib and serve it warm, with the pan juices spooned over the top.

Serving Suggestions:
• Serve the prime rib with roasted potatoes, a fresh salad, and a rich red wine sauce or horseradish cream.
• Offer a selection of condiments, such as horseradish, Dijon mustard, and au jus sauce, for guests to customize their servings.

58. Lobster tails with butter

Ingredient:

- 4 lobster tails, thawed if frozen
- 4 tbsp unsalted butter, melted
- 2 tbsp lemon juice
- 1 tsp garlic powder
- 1/2 tsp paprika
- Salt and pepper to taste

Instructions:

1. Preheat your oven to 400°F (200°C).

2. Using kitchen shears or a sharp knife, carefully cut the top of the lobster tails lengthwise, leaving the bottom shell intact. Gently pull the meat up and out of the shell, leaving the base attached.

3. In a small bowl, whisk together the melted butter, lemon juice, garlic powder, and paprika.

4. Place the lobster tails, meat side up, on a baking sheet or in a baking dish. Brush the lobster meat generously with the butter mixture, making sure to coat it evenly.

5. Season the lobster tails with salt and pepper to taste.

6. Bake the lobster tails for 12•15 minutes, or until the meat is opaque and cooked through.

7. Serve the lobster tails immediately, with the remaining butter mixture drizzled over the top.

Serving Suggestions:

- Serve the lobster tails with lemon wedges, melted butter, or a side of steamed vegetables.

- For a more decadent dish, top the cooked lobster tails with a dollop of hollandaise sauce.

- Pair the lobster tails with a crisp white wine or a light, refreshing cocktail.

59. Pork shoulder roast

Ingredient:

- 4•5 lb pork shoulder roast (also called pork butt)
- 2 tbsp olive oil
- 2 tbsp brown sugar
- 2 tsp salt
- 1 tsp black pepper
- 1 tsp smoked paprika
- 1 tsp garlic powder
- 1 tsp onion powder
- 1 onion, sliced
- 2 cups chicken or beef broth

Instructions:

1. Preheat your oven to 300°F (150°C).

2. In a small bowl, mix together the brown sugar, salt, black pepper, smoked paprika, garlic powder, and onion powder.

3. Rub the pork shoulder all over with the olive oil, then generously coat it with the spice mixture, pressing it into the meat.

4. Place the seasoned pork shoulder in a large roasting pan or Dutch oven. Arrange the sliced onions around the pork.

5. Pour the broth into the bottom of the pan, being careful not to wash off the seasoning on the pork.

6. Cover the pan with a lid or tightly with aluminum foil and roast the pork shoulder for 4•5 hours, or until the meat is very tender and falling apart.

7. Remove the lid or foil during the last 30 minutes of cooking to allow the pork to develop a nice crust.

8. Transfer the roasted pork shoulder to a cutting board and let it rest for 15•20 minutes.Shred or slice the pork and serve it warm, with the cooking juices spooned over the top.

Enjoy your delicious slow•roasted pork shoulder!

60. Lamb rack

Ingredient:

- 1 (8•bone) rack of lamb, frenched (bones exposed)
- 2 tbsp olive oil
- 2 tbsp Dijon mustard
- 2 tbsp chopped fresh rosemary
- 2 tbsp chopped fresh thyme
- 2 garlic cloves, minced
- 1 tsp salt
- 1/2 tsp black pepper

Instructions:

1. Preheat your oven to 400°F (200°C).

2. In a small bowl, mix together the olive oil, Dijon mustard, rosemary, thyme, garlic, salt, and pepper to create a paste.

3. Place the lamb rack, fat side up, on a rimmed baking sheet or in a roasting pan. Generously rub the herb•mustard paste all over the surface of the lamb, making sure to coat the sides and ends as well.

4. Roast the lamb rack for 20•25 minutes for medium•rare doneness (an internal temperature of 130°F/55°C), or 25•30 minutes for medium (an internal temperature of 140°F/60°C).

5. Remove the lamb from the oven and let it rest for 10•15 minutes before slicing.

6. Slice the lamb rack between the bones to create individual chops. Serve the roasted lamb chops warm.

Serving Suggestions:
- Serve the lamb chops with roasted potatoes, a fresh salad, and a drizzle of the pan juices.

- Pair the lamb with a bold red wine, such as a Cabernet Sauvignon or Malbec.

- Garnish the lamb with a sprinkle of chopped fresh parsley or mint.

Enjoy your delicious herb•crusted lamb rack!

61. Beef tenderloin

Ingredient:

- 1 (3•4 lb) beef tenderloin, trimmed
- 2 tbsp olive oil
- 2 tsp salt
- 1 tsp black pepper
- 2 tbsp unsalted butter (optional)

Instructions:

1. Preheat your oven to 450°F (230°C).

2. Pat the beef tenderloin dry with paper towels and rub it all over with the olive oil. Season it generously with the salt and pepper.

3. Place the seasoned tenderloin on a rimmed baking sheet or in a roasting pan.

4. Roast the tenderloin for 40•50 minutes, or until it reaches your desired level of doneness (125°F/52°C for medium•rare, 130°F/54°C for medium).

5. Remove the tenderloin from the oven and let it rest for 15•20 minutes.

6. If desired, top the rested tenderloin with the unsalted butter and let it melt over the hot meat.

7. Slice the beef tenderloin into 1•inch thick slices and serve immediately.

Serving Suggestions:

• Serve the roasted beef tenderloin with roasted potatoes, a fresh salad, and a rich red wine sauce or horseradish cream.

• Offer a selection of condiments, such as Dijon mustard, chimichurri, or a balsamic reduction, for guests to customize their servings.

• Pair the beef tenderloin with a full•bodied red wine, such as a Cabernet Sauvignon or Malbec.

62. Baked chicken thighs

Ingredient:

- 8 bone•in, skin•on chicken thighs
- 2 tbsp olive oil
- 1 tsp salt
- 1/2 tsp black pepper
- 1 tsp paprika
- 1 tsp garlic powder
- 1 tsp dried thyme

Instructions:

1. Preheat your oven to 400°F (200°C). Line a large baking sheet with parchment paper or a silicone baking mat.

2. Pat the chicken thighs dry with paper towels and place them in a large bowl.

3. In a small bowl, mix together the olive oil, salt, black pepper, paprika, garlic powder, and dried thyme.

4. Pour the seasoning mixture over the chicken thighs and toss to coat them evenly.

5. Arrange the seasoned chicken thighs skin•side up on the prepared baking sheet, making sure they are not touching each other.

6. Bake the chicken thighs for 35•40 minutes, or until the skin is crispy and the internal temperature reaches 165°F (75°C).

7. Optionally, you can broil the chicken for 2•3 minutes at the end to further crisp up the skin.

8. Remove the baked chicken thighs from the oven and let them rest for 5 minutes before serving.

Serving Suggestions:

- Serve the crispy baked chicken thighs with roasted vegetables, mashed potatoes, or a fresh salad.

- Top the chicken with a drizzle of honey or a sprinkle of chopped fresh parsley or chives. Pair the chicken thighs with a crisp white wine or a light, refreshing beer.

63. Roasted duck

Ingredient:

- 1 (4.5 lb) whole duck
- 1 tbsp salt
- 1 tsp black pepper
- 1 orange, halved
- 3 sprigs fresh thyme
- 2 garlic cloves, smashed

Instructions:

1. Preheat your oven to 425°F (220°C).

2. Pat the duck dry with paper towels and use a sharp knife to prick small holes all over the skin, being careful not to pierce the meat. This will help the fat render out during cooking.

3. Rub the salt and pepper all over the duck, both inside and out.

4. Place the duck breast•side up on a rack set in a roasting pan. Stuff the cavity with the orange halves, thyme sprigs, and garlic cloves.

5. Roast the duck for 1 hour, then reduce the oven temperature to 350°F (175°C) and continue roasting for an additional 1•1.5 hours, or until the internal temperature of the thigh reaches 165°F (75°C).

6. Baste the duck with the rendered fat in the pan every 30 minutes during the cooking process.

7. Once the duck is cooked, transfer it to a cutting board and let it rest for 15•20 minutes before carving.

8. Carve the duck and serve it warm, with the pan juices spooned over the top.

Serving Suggestions:
• Serve the roasted duck with roasted potatoes, a fresh salad, and a side of cranberry sauce or orange marmalade.
• Use the leftover duck fat to roast vegetables or make crispy roasted potatoes.
• Pair the duck with a full•bodied red wine, such as a Pinot Noir or Malbec.

Enjoy your delicious crispy roasted duck!

64. Goose breast

Ingredient:

- 2 (1•1.5 lb) goose breasts, skin•on
- 1 tsp salt
- 1/2 tsp black pepper
- 1 tbsp olive oil

Instructions:

1. Preheat your oven to 400°F (200°C).

2. Pat the goose breasts dry with paper towels and use a sharp knife to score the skin in a crosshatch pattern, being careful not to cut into the meat.

3. Season the goose breasts all over with the salt and pepper.

4. Heat the olive oil in a large, oven•safe skillet or cast•iron pan over medium•high heat.

5. Place the goose breasts skin•side down in the hot pan and sear for 5•7 minutes, or until the skin is crispy and golden brown.

6. Flip the goose breasts over and transfer the pan to the preheated oven.

7. Roast the goose breasts for 12•15 minutes, or until the internal temperature reaches 135°F (57°C) for medium•rare, or 140°F (60°C) for medium.

8. Remove the pan from the oven and let the goose breasts rest for 5•10 minutes.

9. Slice the roasted goose breasts and serve them warm, with the pan juices spooned over the top.

Serving Suggestions:
- Serve the roasted goose breast with roasted potatoes, a fresh salad, and a side of cranberry sauce or orange marmalade.
- Use the rendered goose fat to roast vegetables or make crispy roasted potatoes.
- Pair the goose with a full•bodied red wine, such as a Pinot Noir or Malbec.

Enjoy your delicious crispy roasted goose breast!

65. Grilled swordfish

Ingredient:

- 4 (6-8 oz) swordfish steaks
- 2 tbsp olive oil
- 1 tsp salt
- 1/2 tsp black pepper
- 1 tbsp lemon juice
- 2 tbsp chopped fresh parsley (optional)

Instructions:

1. Preheat your grill or grill pan to medium-high heat.

2. Pat the swordfish steaks dry with paper towels and brush them all over with the olive oil. Season them evenly with the salt and pepper.

3. Grill the swordfish steaks for 4-5 minutes per side, or until they are opaque and flake easily with a fork.

4. Transfer the grilled swordfish steaks to a serving platter and drizzle them with the lemon juice.

5. If desired, sprinkle the swordfish with the chopped fresh parsley.

6. Serve the grilled swordfish steaks immediately, while hot.

Serving Suggestions:

- Serve the grilled swordfish with roasted vegetables, a fresh salad, or a side of grilled lemon slices.

- Top the swordfish with a dollop of pesto, a drizzle of balsamic reduction, or a sprinkle of toasted breadcrumbs.

- Pair the grilled swordfish with a crisp white wine, such as a Sauvignon Blanc or Pinot Grigio.

Enjoy your delicious grilled swordfish!

66. Smoked pork belly

Ingredient:

- 3•4 lb pork belly, skin on
- 2 tbsp brown sugar
- 2 tsp salt
- 1 tsp black pepper
- 1 tsp smoked paprika
- 1 tsp garlic powder
- 1 tsp onion powder
- Wood chips for smoking (such as apple, hickory, or mesquite)

Instructions:

1. Pat the pork belly dry with paper towels and place it on a cutting board. Use a sharp knife to score the skin in a crosshatch pattern, making sure not to cut too deep into the meat.

2. In a small bowl, mix together the brown sugar, salt, black pepper, smoked paprika, garlic powder, and onion powder. Rub the seasoning mixture all over the pork belly, including the scored skin.

3. Prepare your smoker according to the manufacturer's instructions. Soak the wood chips in water for 30 minutes before adding them to the smoker.

4. Place the seasoned pork belly, skin•side up, on the grill grates of the smoker. Close the lid and smoke the pork belly for 4•6 hours, or until the internal temperature reaches 195°F (91°C).

5. During the smoking process, replenish the wood chips as needed to maintain a steady stream of smoke.

6. Once the pork belly is fully cooked, remove it from the smoker and let it rest for 15•20 minutes.

7. Slice the smoked pork belly and serve it warm, with any desired sauces or accompaniments.

Tips:
- For extra crispy skin, you can broil the pork belly for 2•3 minutes after smoking.
- Adjust the smoking time as needed, depending on the thickness of your pork belly and your desired level of doneness.

67. Osso buco (without vegetables)

Ingredient:

- 1 cup beef or veal stock
- 1 (14.5 oz) can diced tomatoes
- 2 bay leaves
- 2 sprigs fresh thyme
- 1 tsp salt
- 1/2 tsp black pepper

- 4 (1•inch thick) veal osso buco shanks
- 2 tbsp olive oil
- 1 onion, diced
- 3 garlic cloves, minced
- 1 cup dry white wine

Instructions:

1. Pat the veal osso buco shanks dry with paper towels and season them all over with the salt and pepper.

2. Heat the olive oil in a large, heavy•bottomed pot or Dutch oven over medium•high heat.

3. Working in batches if needed, sear the veal shanks on all sides until they are golden brown, about 3•4 minutes per side. Transfer the seared shanks to a plate.

4. Reduce the heat to medium and add the diced onion to the pot. Cook, stirring occasionally, until the onion is softened and translucent, about 5 minutes.

5. Add the minced garlic and cook for an additional minute, until fragrant.

6. Pour in the white wine and use a wooden spoon to scrape up any browned bits from the bottom of the pot.

7. Add the diced tomatoes, beef or veal stock, bay leaves, and thyme sprigs. Bring the mixture to a simmer.

8. Return the seared veal shanks to the pot, cover, and transfer to a preheated 325°F (165°C) oven.

9. Braise the osso buco in the oven for 2•2.5 hours, or until the meat is very tender and falling off the bone.

10. Remove the pot from the oven and transfer the veal shanks to a serving platter. Discard the bay leaves and thyme sprigs.

68. Leg of lamb

Ingredient:

- 4•5 lb leg of lamb, bone•in or boneless
- 3 cloves garlic, minced
- 2 tbsp fresh rosemary, chopped
- 2 tsp salt
- 1 tsp black pepper
- 2 tbsp olive oil

Instructions:

1. Preheat your oven to 450°F (230°C).

2. In a small bowl, mix together the minced garlic, chopped rosemary, salt, and pepper.

3. Rub the garlic•herb mixture all over the surface of the lamb leg, making sure to coat it evenly.

4. Drizzle the olive oil over the lamb and rub it in to help the seasoning adhere.

5. Place the lamb in a roasting pan or on a rimmed baking sheet.

6. Roast the lamb for 15 minutes at 450°F, then reduce the temperature to 325°F (165°C) and continue roasting until it reaches your desired doneness, about 1•1.5 hours for medium•rare.

7. Use a meat thermometer to check the internal temperature. For medium•rare, aim for 130•135°F. For medium, 140•145°F.

8. Once cooked, let the lamb rest for 10•15 minutes before slicing and serving.

Enjoy your delicious roasted leg of lamb!

69. Grilled mahi•mahi

Ingredient:

• 4 mahi•mahi fillets (about 6 oz each)
• 2 tbsp olive oil
• 2 tsp lemon juice
• 1 tsp garlic powder
• 1 tsp paprika
• 1 tsp dried oregano
• 1 tsp salt
• 1/2 tsp black pepper

Instructions:

1. Preheat your grill to medium•high heat.

2. In a shallow dish, combine the olive oil, lemon juice, garlic powder, paprika, oregano, salt, and pepper. Mix well.

3. Add the mahi•mahi fillets to the dish and turn to coat both sides evenly with the seasoning mixture.

4. Grill the mahi•mahi for 4•5 minutes per side, or until the fish flakes easily with a fork and reaches an internal temperature of 145°F.

5. Transfer the grilled mahi•mahi fillets to a serving platter.

6. Serve the grilled mahi•mahi immediately, garnished with lemon wedges if desired.

Tips:
• Be careful not to overcook the mahi•mahi, as it can become dry and tough.
• You can also use this seasoning blend for baked or pan•seared mahi•mahi.
• Mahi•mahi is a firm, mild•flavored fish that pairs well with a variety of seasonings and sauces.

Enjoy your delicious grilled mahi•mahi!

70. Beef tongue

Ingredient:

- 1 beef tongue, about 2•3 lbs
- 1 onion, diced
- 3 carrots, peeled and diced
- 3 celery stalks, diced
- 4 garlic cloves, minced
- 2 bay leaves
- 1 tsp black peppercorns
- 1 tsp salt
- 4 cups beef broth or water

Instructions:

1. Rinse the beef tongue under cold water and place it in a large pot. Cover with water and bring to a boil over high heat.

2. Reduce the heat to medium•low, cover the pot, and simmer the tongue for 2•3 hours, or until it is very tender and the skin can be easily peeled off.

3. Drain the tongue and let it cool slightly. Once it's cool enough to handle, peel off the skin and discard it.

4. In a large Dutch oven or heavy•bottomed pot, combine the peeled tongue, onion, carrots, celery, garlic, bay leaves, peppercorns, and salt. Pour in the beef broth or water, making sure the tongue is fully submerged.

5. Bring the mixture to a boil, then reduce the heat to low, cover the pot, and simmer for 2•3 hours, or until the tongue is very tender and easily shreds with a fork.

6. Remove the bay leaves. Using two forks, shred or slice the beef tongue.

7. Serve the braised beef tongue warm, with the cooking liquid spooned over the top. Adjust the seasoning with salt and pepper to taste.

Serving Suggestions:
- Serve the braised beef tongue on sandwiches, tacos, or over mashed potatoes.
- Use the shredded tongue in stews, chili, or as a topping for nachos.
- Garnish the tongue with chopped onions, cilantro, or a drizzle of chimichurri sauce.

71. Pork schnitzel (no breading)

Ingredient:

- 4 boneless pork chops, pounded thin (about 1/4 inch thick)
- 2 tbsp olive oil
- 2 tbsp butter
- 1 tsp garlic powder
- 1 tsp paprika
- 1 tsp salt
- 1/2 tsp black pepper

Instructions:

1. Prepare the pork chops: Place the pork chops between two sheets of plastic wrap or parchment paper and pound them with a meat mallet or the bottom of a heavy pan until they are about 1/4 inch thick.

2. In a shallow bowl, mix together the garlic powder, paprika, salt, and black pepper.

3. Coat both sides of the pounded pork chops with the seasoning mixture, pressing it in gently to adhere.

4. Heat the olive oil and butter in a large skillet over medium•high heat.

5. When the oil and butter are hot, add the seasoned pork chops to the skillet in a single layer. You may need to work in batches depending on the size of your skillet.

6. Cook the pork chops for 2•3 minutes per side, or until they are golden brown and cooked through. The internal temperature should reach 145°F.

7. Transfer the cooked pork schnitzel to a plate and let them rest for a few minutes before serving.

Serve the pork schnitzel hot, garnished with lemon wedges if desired. You can also serve it with your favorite sides, such as roasted potatoes, sautéed vegetables, or a fresh salad.

Enjoy your delicious pork schnitzel without the breading!

72. Chicken fried steak (using pork rinds for breading)

Ingredient:

- 4 thin•cut beef steaks (such as cube steak or tenderized round steak)
- 1 cup crushed pork rinds
- 1 tsp garlic powder
- 1 tsp onion powder
- 1 tsp paprika
- 1 tsp salt
- 1/2 tsp black pepper
- 2 eggs, beaten
- 2 tbsp milk
- Vegetable oil for frying

For the Gravy:
- 2 tbsp butter
- 2 tbsp all•purpose flour
- 2 cups milk
- 1 tsp salt
- 1/4 tsp black pepper

Instructions:

1. Prepare the steaks: Pound the beef steaks between two sheets of plastic wrap or parchment paper until they are about 1/4 inch thick.

2. In a shallow bowl, mix together the crushed pork rinds, garlic powder, onion powder, paprika, salt, and black pepper.

3. In a separate shallow bowl, whisk together the beaten eggs and milk.

4. Dip the pounded beef steaks into the egg mixture, allowing any excess to drip off. Then dredge the steaks in the pork rind breading, pressing it in to help it adhere.

5. In a large skillet, heat about 1/4 inch of vegetable oil over medium•high heat.

6. Carefully add the breaded steaks to the hot oil and fry for 3•4 minutes per side, or until golden brown and cooked through. Transfer the fried steaks to a paper towel•lined plate.

For the Gravy:
1. In the same skillet, melt the butter over medium heat. Whisk in the flour and cook for 1•2 minutes, stirring constantly.

2. Gradually whisk in the milk and cook, stirring frequently, until the gravy thickens, about 5•7 minutes.

3. Season the gravy with salt and pepper.

73. Baked cod fillet

Ingredient:

- 4 cod fillets (about 6 oz each)
- 2 tbsp olive oil
- 2 tbsp lemon juice
- 1 tsp garlic powder
- 1 tsp paprika
- 1 tsp dried parsley
- 1/2 tsp salt
- 1/4 tsp black pepper

Instructions:

1. Preheat your oven to 400°F (200°C).

2. Pat the cod fillets dry with paper towels and place them in a baking dish or on a rimmed baking sheet.

3. In a small bowl, whisk together the olive oil, lemon juice, garlic powder, paprika, dried parsley, salt, and black pepper.

4. Drizzle the seasoning mixture over the cod fillets, making sure to evenly coat the top and sides of the fish.

5. Bake the cod in the preheated oven for 12•15 minutes, or until the fish flakes easily with a fork and reaches an internal temperature of 145°F (63°C).

6. Remove the baked cod from the oven and let it rest for a few minutes.

7. Serve the baked cod fillets hot, garnished with additional lemon wedges if desired.

Tips:
- You can use other types of white fish, such as halibut or tilapia, in this recipe.
- For extra flavor, you can add some chopped fresh herbs, such as dill or parsley, to the seasoning mixture.
- Bake the cod on a parchment•lined baking sheet for easier cleanup.

74. Wild boar ribs

Ingredient:

- 2 lbs wild boar ribs, cut into individual ribs
- 1/4 cup brown sugar
- 2 tbsp smoked paprika
- 2 tsp garlic powder
- 2 tsp onion powder
- 1 tsp salt
- 1 tsp black pepper
- 1/4 cup apple cider vinegar
- 2 tbsp Dijon mustard
- 2 tbsp honey

For the Sauce:
- 1 cup ketchup
- 1/4 cup apple cider vinegar
- 2 tbsp brown sugar
- 1 tbsp Worcestershire sauce
- 1 tsp smoked paprika
- 1/2 tsp garlic powder
- 1/2 tsp onion powder
- 1/4 tsp cayenne pepper (optional)

Instructions:

1. In a small bowl, mix together the brown sugar, smoked paprika, garlic powder, onion powder, salt, and black pepper. Rub this seasoning mixture all over the wild boar ribs.

2. In a separate bowl, whisk together the apple cider vinegar, Dijon mustard, and honey. Pour this mixture over the seasoned ribs and toss to coat.

3. Cover the ribs and refrigerate for at least 2 hours, or up to 24 hours, to allow the flavors to develop.

4. Preheat your grill to medium•high heat.

5. Grill the ribs for 20•25 minutes, turning occasionally, until they are lightly charred and cooked through.

For the Sauce:
1. In a small saucepan, combine all the sauce ingredients and bring to a simmer over medium heat.

2. Reduce the heat and let the sauce simmer for 10•15 minutes, stirring occasionally, until thickened.

Serve the grilled wild boar ribs hot, with the homemade barbecue sauce on the side for dipping or drizzling over the top.

75. Grilled octopus

Ingredient:

- 1 lb octopus, cleaned and tentacles separated
- 2 tbsp olive oil
- 2 tbsp lemon juice
- 2 cloves garlic, minced
- 1 tsp dried oregano
- 1 tsp paprika
- 1/2 tsp salt
- 1/4 tsp black pepper

Instructions:

1. In a large bowl, combine the olive oil, lemon juice, garlic, oregano, paprika, salt, and black pepper. Add the octopus tentacles and toss to coat them evenly in the marinade.

2. Cover the bowl and refrigerate the marinated octopus for at least 30 minutes, up to 2 hours.

3. Preheat your grill to medium•high heat.

4. Remove the octopus from the marinade and thread the tentacles onto skewers, leaving a little space between each piece.

5. Grill the octopus skewers for 3•5 minutes per side, or until the octopus is lightly charred and cooked through. The tentacles should be tender but still have a slight bite to them.

6. Transfer the grilled octopus skewers to a serving platter. Drizzle any remaining marinade over the top.

7. Serve the grilled octopus warm, garnished with lemon wedges if desired.

Tips:
- Look for fresh, high•quality octopus for the best results.
- You can also grill the octopus without skewers, but skewers make it easier to handle.
- Adjust the grilling time based on the thickness of your octopus tentacles.

76. Turkey leg

Ingredient:

- 2 whole turkey legs (drumstick and thigh)
- 2 tbsp olive oil
- 2 tsp salt
- 1 tsp black pepper
- 1 tsp garlic powder
- 1 tsp dried thyme
- 1 tsp dried rosemary
- 1/2 tsp smoked paprika

Instructions:

1. Preheat your oven to 375°F (190°C).

2. Pat the turkey legs dry with paper towels and place them in a large baking dish or on a rimmed baking sheet.

3. In a small bowl, mix together the olive oil, salt, black pepper, garlic powder, dried thyme, dried rosemary, and smoked paprika.

4. Rub the seasoning mixture all over the turkey legs, making sure to coat them evenly.

5. Roast the turkey legs in the preheated oven for 1 to 1.5 hours, or until the internal temperature reaches 165°F (74°C) when measured with a meat thermometer.

6. Baste the turkey legs with the pan juices a few times during the roasting process to keep them moist.

7. Once the turkey legs are cooked through, remove them from the oven and let them rest for 5•10 minutes before serving.

Serve the roasted turkey legs hot, with the pan juices spooned over the top. You can also serve them with your favorite sides, such as roasted vegetables, mashed potatoes, or a fresh salad.

77. Venison chili (meat only)

Ingredient:

- 2 lbs ground venison
- 2 tbsp olive oil
- 1 large onion, diced
- 3 cloves garlic, minced
- 2 tbsp chili powder
- 2 tsp ground cumin
- 1 tsp dried oregano
- 1 tsp smoked paprika
- 1 tsp salt
- 1/2 tsp black pepper
- 1/4 tsp cayenne pepper (optional, for more heat)
- 1 (14.5 oz) can diced tomatoes
- 1 cup beef or chicken broth

Toppings (optional):
- Shredded cheddar cheese
- Sour cream
- Chopped green onions
- Diced avocado

Instructions:

1. In a large pot or Dutch oven, heat the olive oil over medium•high heat. Add the ground venison and cook, breaking it up with a wooden spoon, until browned, about 5•7 minutes.

2. Add the diced onion and minced garlic to the pot. Cook for 2•3 minutes, stirring frequently, until the onion is translucent.

3. Stir in the chili powder, cumin, oregano, smoked paprika, salt, black pepper, and cayenne (if using). Cook for 1 minute to toast the spices.

4. Pour in the diced tomatoes and beef or chicken broth. Stir to combine.

5. Bring the chili to a simmer, then reduce the heat to low. Let the chili simmer, uncovered, for 30•45 minutes, stirring occasionally, until the flavors have melded and the chili has thickened.

6. Taste and adjust seasoning as needed, adding more salt, pepper, or spices to your preference.

7. Serve the venison chili hot, topped with shredded cheddar cheese, sour cream, chopped green onions, and/or diced avocado, if desired.

78. Rabbit stew (meat only)

Ingredient:

- 2 lbs rabbit meat, cut into 1·inch pieces
- 2 tbsp olive oil
- 1 onion, diced
- 3 cloves garlic, minced
- 2 tbsp all·purpose flour
- 2 cups chicken or beef broth
- 1 cup dry white wine
- 2 tsp dried thyme
- 1 tsp dried rosemary
- 1 tsp salt
- 1/2 tsp black pepper

Instructions:

1. In a large Dutch oven or heavy·bottomed pot, heat the olive oil over medium·high heat.

2. Add the rabbit meat to the pot and brown it on all sides, about 5·7 minutes. Transfer the browned rabbit to a plate and set aside.

3. Reduce the heat to medium and add the diced onion to the pot. Cook the onion for 3·4 minutes, stirring frequently, until it starts to soften.

4. Add the minced garlic to the pot and cook for 1 minute, until fragrant.

5. Sprinkle the all·purpose flour over the onions and garlic. Stir to coat and cook for 1 minute.

6. Gradually whisk in the chicken or beef broth and the white wine. Bring the liquid to a simmer.

7. Return the browned rabbit meat to the pot and add the dried thyme, dried rosemary, salt, and black pepper.

8. Reduce the heat to low, cover the pot, and let the stew simmer for 45·60 minutes, or until the rabbit meat is very tender.

9. Taste the stew and adjust the seasoning as needed, adding more salt, pepper, or herbs to your preference.

79. BBQ beef ribs

Ingredient:

- 3 lbs beef short ribs, cut into individual ribs
- 2 tbsp brown sugar
- 2 tsp smoked paprika
- 1 tsp garlic powder
- 1 tsp onion powder
- 1 tsp salt
- 1/2 tsp black pepper
- 1/4 cup apple cider vinegar
- 1 cup barbecue sauce (your favorite brand or homemade)

Instructions:

1. Preheat your grill to medium•high heat, about 375•400°F (190•205°C).

2. In a small bowl, mix together the brown sugar, smoked paprika, garlic powder, onion powder, salt, and black pepper.

3. Generously rub the seasoning mixture all over the beef short ribs, making sure to coat them evenly on all sides.

4. Place the seasoned ribs on the preheated grill and cook for 30•40 minutes, turning occasionally, until they are lightly charred and starting to become tender.

5. In a small bowl, whisk together the apple cider vinegar and barbecue sauce.

6. Brush the ribs with the barbecue sauce mixture, then continue grilling for an additional 15•20 minutes, turning and basting with the sauce occasionally, until the ribs are cooked through and the sauce has caramelized.

7. Transfer the grilled BBQ beef ribs to a serving platter. Let them rest for 5•10 minutes before serving.

8. Serve the BBQ beef ribs hot, with any remaining sauce on the side for dipping or drizzling over the top.

Tips:
- You can also finish the ribs in the oven at 375°F (190°C) for 30•45 minutes if you don't want to grill them.

80. Frog legs

Ingredient:

- 1 lb frog legs, cleaned and patted dry
- 1 cup all•purpose flour
- 1 tsp salt
- 1/2 tsp black pepper
- 1/2 tsp paprika
- Vegetable oil for frying

For Serving (optional):
- Lemon wedges
- Tartar sauce or remoulade sauce

Instructions:

1. In a shallow bowl, mix together the flour, salt, black pepper, and paprika.

2. Working in batches, dredge the frog legs in the seasoned flour, making sure to coat them evenly on all sides.

3. In a large skillet or Dutch oven, heat about 1•2 inches of vegetable oil over medium•high heat to 350°F (175°C).

4. Carefully add the floured frog legs to the hot oil and fry for 3•5 minutes per side, or until golden brown and crispy.

5. Use a slotted spoon or tongs to transfer the fried frog legs to a paper towel•lined plate to drain any excess oil.

6. Serve the fried frog legs hot, with lemon wedges and tartar sauce or remoulade sauce on the side, if desired.

Tips:
- Make sure to clean and pat the frog legs dry before breading to help the flour adhere.
- Adjust the frying time based on the size of your frog legs. Smaller pieces may cook faster.
- You can also bake the breaded frog legs at 400°F (200°C) for 15•20 minutes, flipping halfway, for a healthier alternative to frying.

81. Elk steak

Ingredient:

- 2 elk steaks (about 8 oz each)
- 2 tbsp olive oil
- 2 tsp garlic powder
- 2 tsp dried oregano
- 1 tsp salt
- 1/2 tsp black pepper

Instructions:

1. Pat the elk steaks dry with paper towels and place them in a shallow dish or resealable bag.

2. In a small bowl, mix together the olive oil, garlic powder, dried oregano, salt, and black pepper.

3. Pour the seasoning mixture over the elk steaks and rub it in to coat both sides evenly.

4. Cover the dish or seal the bag and let the steaks marinate in the refrigerator for 30 minutes to 1 hour.

5. Preheat your grill to medium•high heat, about 400•450°F (200•230°C).

6. Grill the elk steaks for 3•5 minutes per side, or until they reach your desired level of doneness. For medium•rare, aim for an internal temperature of 130•135°F (54•57°C).

7. Transfer the grilled elk steaks to a cutting board and let them rest for 5•10 minutes before slicing and serving.

Serve the grilled elk steak hot, garnished with additional fresh oregano or parsley if desired. You can also serve it with your favorite sides, such as roasted vegetables or a fresh salad.

Tips:
- Elk is a lean meat, so be careful not to overcook it to keep it tender and juicy.
- You can also pan•sear the elk steaks in a hot skillet instead of grilling them.
- Adjust the cooking time based on the thickness of your elk steaks.

82. Roast quail

Ingredient:

- 4 whole quail, patted dry
- 2 tbsp olive oil
- 1 tsp salt
- 1/2 tsp black pepper
- 1/2 tsp dried thyme
- 1/2 tsp dried rosemary
- 2 cloves garlic, minced
- 1/4 cup dry white wine or chicken broth

Instructions:

1. Preheat your oven to 400°F (200°C).

2. In a small bowl, mix together the olive oil, salt, black pepper, dried thyme, dried rosemary, and minced garlic.

3. Rub the seasoning mixture all over the quail, making sure to coat them evenly.

4. Place the seasoned quail in a baking dish or on a rimmed baking sheet. Pour the white wine or chicken broth into the bottom of the dish.

5. Roast the quail in the preheated oven for 25•30 minutes, or until the internal temperature reaches 165°F (74°C) when measured with a meat thermometer.

6. Baste the quail with the pan juices a few times during the roasting process to keep them moist.

7. Once the quail are cooked, remove them from the oven and let them rest for 5•10 minutes before serving.

Serve the roasted quail hot, with the pan juices spooned over the top. You can also garnish them with fresh thyme or rosemary sprigs.

Tips:
- Quail is a small, delicate bird, so be careful not to overcook it.
- You can also grill the quail instead of roasting them in the oven.
- Adjust the cooking time based on the size of your quail.

83. Seared ahi tuna

Ingredient:

- 4 (6 oz) ahi tuna steaks
- 2 tbsp sesame oil
- 2 tbsp soy sauce
- 1 tbsp honey
- 1 tsp grated ginger
- 1 tsp sesame seeds
- 1/2 tsp black pepper

Instructions:

1. In a shallow dish, whisk together the sesame oil, soy sauce, honey, grated ginger, sesame seeds, and black pepper.

2. Add the ahi tuna steaks to the dish and turn to coat them evenly in the marinade. Cover and refrigerate for 30 minutes to 1 hour.

3. Heat a large skillet or grill pan over high heat.

4. Remove the tuna steaks from the marinade and pat them dry with paper towels.

5. Sear the tuna steaks for 1•2 minutes per side, or until the outside is lightly charred but the center is still rare to medium•rare.

6. Transfer the seared ahi tuna steaks to a cutting board and let them rest for 2•3 minutes.

7. Slice the tuna steaks across the grain into 1/2•inch thick slices.

Serve the seared ahi tuna slices immediately, drizzled with any remaining marinade from the dish. You can also serve it with steamed rice, a fresh salad, or your favorite Asian•inspired sides.

Tips:
- Look for the freshest, sushi•grade ahi tuna for the best results.
- Be careful not to overcook the tuna, as it's best enjoyed rare to medium•rare.
- You can also sear the tuna on a very hot grill for a similar effect.

84. Pheasant breast

Ingredient:

- 2 pheasant breasts, bone•in and skin•on
- 2 tbsp olive oil
- 1 tsp salt
- 1/2 tsp black pepper
- 1 tsp dried thyme
- 1 tsp dried rosemary
- 2 cloves garlic, minced
- 1/2 cup dry white wine or chicken broth

Instructions:

1. Preheat your oven to 400°F (200°C).

2. Pat the pheasant breasts dry with paper towels and place them in a baking dish or on a rimmed baking sheet.

3. In a small bowl, mix together the olive oil, salt, black pepper, dried thyme, dried rosemary, and minced garlic.

4. Rub the seasoning mixture all over the pheasant breasts, making sure to coat the skin and any exposed meat.

5. Pour the white wine or chicken broth into the bottom of the baking dish or sheet.

6. Roast the pheasant breasts in the preheated oven for 25•30 minutes, or until the internal temperature reaches 160°F (71°C) when measured with a meat thermometer.

7. Remove the roasted pheasant breasts from the oven and let them rest for 5•10 minutes before slicing and serving.

8. Optionally, you can baste the pheasant with the pan juices a few times during the roasting process to keep it moist.

Serve the roasted pheasant breast hot, with the pan juices spooned over the top. You can also serve it with your favorite sides, such as roasted vegetables or a fresh salad.

85. Lamb liver

Ingredient:

- 1 lb lamb liver, trimmed and sliced into 1/4•inch thick pieces
- 2 tbsp olive oil
- 1 onion, thinly sliced
- 3 cloves garlic, minced
- 1 tsp dried thyme
- 1 tsp salt
- 1/2 tsp black pepper
- 1/4 cup dry white wine or chicken broth

Instructions:

1. Pat the lamb liver slices dry with paper towels and season them with salt and pepper.

2. In a large skillet, heat the olive oil over medium•high heat.

3. Working in batches if needed, add the seasoned lamb liver slices to the hot skillet and sauté for 2•3 minutes per side, or until they are lightly browned on the outside but still slightly pink in the center.

4. Transfer the sautéed liver to a plate and set aside.

5. Reduce the heat to medium and add the sliced onion to the skillet. Sauté the onion for 3•4 minutes, until it starts to soften.

6. Add the minced garlic and dried thyme to the skillet and cook for 1 minute, until fragrant.

7. Pour in the white wine or chicken broth and use a wooden spoon to scrape up any browned bits from the bottom of the skillet.

8. Return the sautéed lamb liver to the skillet and let the mixture simmer for 2•3 minutes, until the sauce has thickened slightly.

9. Taste and adjust the seasoning as needed, adding more salt and pepper if desired.

Serve the sautéed lamb liver hot, garnished with additional thyme sprigs if desired. It pairs well with mashed potatoes, roasted vegetables, or a fresh salad.

86. Beef jerky

Ingredient:

- 2 lbs beef sirloin or flank steak, thinly sliced against the grain
- 1/4 cup soy sauce
- 2 tbsp Worcestershire sauce
- 2 tbsp brown sugar
- 2 tsp smoked paprika
- 1 tsp garlic powder
- 1 tsp onion powder
- 1 tsp black pepper
- 1/2 tsp red pepper flakes (optional, for spicy jerky)

Instructions:

1. In a large resealable bag or bowl, combine the soy sauce, Worcestershire sauce, brown sugar, smoked paprika, garlic powder, onion powder, black pepper, and red pepper flakes (if using). Mix well.

2. Add the sliced beef to the marinade and toss to coat the meat evenly. Cover or seal the bag and refrigerate for 4·6 hours, or up to 24 hours, turning the bag occasionally.

3. Preheat your oven to the lowest setting, usually around 135·145°F (57·63°C). Line 2·3 baking sheets with parchment paper or silicone baking mats.

4. Remove the beef slices from the marinade and pat them dry with paper towels. Arrange the beef slices in a single layer on the prepared baking sheets, making sure they don't overlap.

5. Place the baking sheets in the preheated oven and let the beef jerky dry for 4·6 hours, or until it reaches your desired level of dryness. Flip the beef slices halfway through the drying process.

6. Once the jerky is done, remove it from the oven and let it cool completely before storing.

7. Store the beef jerky in an airtight container at room temperature for up to 2 weeks, or in the refrigerator for up to 1 month.

87. Pork rinds

Ingredient:

• 1 lb pork skin, with fat attached
• Vegetable oil for frying
• Salt

Instructions:

1. Rinse the pork skin under cold water and pat it dry with paper towels. Use a sharp knife to trim off any excess fat, leaving about 1/4 inch of fat attached to the skin.

2. Cut the pork skin into 1•inch wide strips.

3. In a large, heavy•bottomed pot or Dutch oven, heat 2•3 inches of vegetable oil to 375°F (190°C).

4. Working in batches, carefully add the pork skin strips to the hot oil. Fry for 3•5 minutes, or until the pork rinds have puffed up and turned golden brown.

5. Use a slotted spoon or tongs to transfer the fried pork rinds to a paper towel•lined plate or baking sheet.

6. Immediately season the hot pork rinds generously with salt.

7. Allow the pork rinds to cool completely before serving.

Tips:
• For best results, use fresh, uncured pork skin. Avoid using skin that has been cured or smoked.
• Make sure the oil is hot enough before adding the pork skin. The temperature should remain between 350•375°F (177•190°C) during frying.
• Fry the pork skin in small batches to maintain the oil temperature and ensure even cooking.
• For extra flavor, you can season the pork rinds with other spices, such as garlic powder, onion powder, or chili powder.
• Store the cooled pork rinds in an airtight container at room temperature for up to 1 week.

88. Cheese crisps

Ingredient:

- 1 cup shredded cheddar cheese
- 1/4 cup shredded Parmesan cheese
- 1/4 tsp garlic powder (optional)
- 1/4 tsp paprika (optional)

Instructions:

1. Preheat your oven to 375°F (190°C). Line a baking sheet with parchment paper.

2. In a small bowl, mix together the shredded cheddar cheese, shredded Parmesan cheese, garlic powder (if using), and paprika (if using) until well combined.

3. Scoop tablespoon·sized portions of the cheese mixture onto the prepared baking sheet, spacing them about 2 inches apart.

4. Use the back of a spoon or your fingers to gently flatten and shape the cheese portions into thin, round discs.

5. Bake the cheese crisps in the preheated oven for 8·10 minutes, or until they are golden brown and crispy.

6. Remove the baking sheet from the oven and let the cheese crisps cool on the sheet for 2·3 minutes before transferring them to a wire rack to cool completely.

7. Once cooled, the cheese crisps should be crisp and ready to serve.

Tips:
- You can use a variety of shredded cheeses, such as cheddar, Parmesan, Gruyère, or Gouda, to create different flavors.

- Experiment with different spices and seasonings, like cayenne pepper, smoked paprika, or dried herbs, to add more flavor.

- Make sure the cheese crisps are spaced apart on the baking sheet to allow for even cooking and crisping.

- Store the cooled cheese crisps in an airtight container at room temperature for up to 1 week.

89. Hard•boiled eggs

Ingredient:

• 6 large eggs

Instructions:

1. Place the eggs in a single layer in a saucepan and cover with cold water by 1 inch.

2. Bring the water to a boil over high heat. Once the water reaches a rolling boil, remove the pan from the heat and cover with a lid.

3. Let the eggs sit in the hot water for the following times, depending on your desired doneness:
   • For soft•boiled eggs: 6•7 minutes
   • For hard•boiled eggs: 12 minutes

4. Drain the hot water and cover the eggs with cold water. Let them sit in the cold water for 5 minutes.

5. Gently tap the eggs against the counter to crack the shells, then peel them starting from the wider end of the egg.

6. Rinse the peeled eggs under cold water to remove any remaining shell fragments.

7. Serve the hard•boiled eggs as desired, or refrigerate them in an airtight container for up to 1 week.

Tips:
• Use eggs that are at least a week old, as they are easier to peel.

• Add a teaspoon of baking soda to the cooking water to help the shells release more easily.

• Shock the cooked eggs in an ice bath to stop the cooking process and make them easier to peel.

• For a more tender yolk, reduce the cooking time by a minute or two.

90. Smoked salmon slices

Ingredient:

- 8 oz thinly sliced smoked salmon
- 1 tbsp capers, drained
- 1 tbsp finely chopped red onion
- 1 tbsp chopped fresh dill (or 1 tsp dried dill)
- 1 tbsp lemon juice
- 1/4 tsp black pepper

Serving Suggestions:
- Crackers or toasted bread
- Cream cheese
- Sliced cucumber or tomato
- Lemon wedges

Instructions:

1. In a small bowl, gently mix together the sliced smoked salmon, capers, red onion, fresh dill (or dried dill), lemon juice, and black pepper.

2. Arrange the smoked salmon mixture on a serving platter or plate.

3. Serve the smoked salmon slices with your desired accompaniments, such as crackers, toasted bread, cream cheese, sliced cucumber or tomato, and lemon wedges.

Tips:
- Use high•quality, thinly sliced smoked salmon for the best flavor and texture.
- Adjust the amounts of capers, onion, dill, and lemon juice to suit your taste preferences.
- For a creamier presentation, you can mix the smoked salmon with a small amount of softened cream cheese before serving.
- Garnish the platter with additional fresh dill sprigs or lemon wedges for a nice visual appeal.
- Serve the smoked salmon slices chilled or at room temperature.

91. Pepperoni sticks

Ingredient:

- 1 lb ground pork
- 2 tsp salt
- 1 tsp black pepper
- 1 tsp paprika
- 1 tsp garlic powder
- 1 tsp onion powder
- 1/2 tsp red pepper flakes (optional, for spicy pepperoni)
- 1/4 tsp curing salt (such as Prague Powder #1)

Instructions:

1. In a large bowl, combine the ground pork, salt, black pepper, paprika, garlic powder, onion powder, red pepper flakes (if using), and curing salt. Mix well until the seasonings are evenly distributed.

2. Divide the seasoned pork mixture into 8 equal portions. Roll each portion into a long, thin stick, about 1/2 inch in diameter and 6-8 inches long.

3. Place the pepperoni sticks on a baking sheet or plate and refrigerate for at least 2 hours, or up to 24 hours, to allow the flavors to develop.

4. Preheat your oven to 225°F (110°C).

5. Line a baking sheet with parchment paper or a silicone baking mat.

6. Arrange the chilled pepperoni sticks on the prepared baking sheet, spacing them about 1 inch apart.

7. Bake the pepperoni sticks in the preheated oven for 2-3 hours, or until they are firm and dry to the touch.

8. Remove the baked pepperoni sticks from the oven and let them cool completely.

9. Once cooled, you can wrap the pepperoni sticks individually in plastic wrap or parchment paper for storage.

Store the homemade pepperoni sticks in the refrigerator for up to 2 weeks, or in the freezer for up to 3 months.

92. Chicken liver bites

Ingredient:

- 1 lb chicken livers, trimmed and cut into 1•inch pieces
- 1/2 cup all•purpose flour
- 1 tsp salt
- 1/2 tsp black pepper
- 1/2 tsp paprika
- 2 tbsp olive oil
- 2 tbsp butter

For Serving (optional):
- Lemon wedges
- Chopped parsley

Instructions:

1. In a shallow bowl, combine the all•purpose flour, salt, black pepper, and paprika. Mix well.

2. Dredge the chicken liver pieces in the seasoned flour, making sure to coat them evenly on all sides.

3. In a large skillet, heat the olive oil and butter over medium•high heat.

4. Working in batches if needed, add the floured chicken liver pieces to the hot skillet and sauté for 2•3 minutes per side, or until they are golden brown and cooked through.

5. Transfer the sautéed chicken liver bites to a paper towel•lined plate to drain any excess oil. Serve the chicken liver bites hot, garnished with lemon wedges and chopped parsley, if desired.

Tips:
- Make sure to trim any connective tissue or discolored parts from the chicken livers before cooking.

- Adjust the cooking time based on the size of your chicken liver pieces. Smaller pieces may cook faster.

- You can also bake the chicken liver bites at 400°F (200°C) for 15•20 minutes, turning halfway, for a healthier alternative to frying.

93. Bacon strips

Ingredient:

• 12 oz thick•cut bacon slices

Instructions:

1. Preheat your oven to 400°F (200°C). Line a large baking sheet with parchment paper or a silicone baking mat.

2. Arrange the bacon slices in a single layer on the prepared baking sheet, making sure they don't overlap.

3. Bake the bacon in the preheated oven for 15•20 minutes, or until it is crispy and golden brown.

4. Flip the bacon slices halfway through the cooking time to ensure even crisping.

5. Once the bacon is cooked to your desired level of crispiness, remove the baking sheet from the oven.

6. Use tongs or a slotted spoon to transfer the crispy bacon strips to a paper towel•lined plate to drain any excess grease.

7. Serve the bacon strips hot, or let them cool completely before storing.

Tips:
• For extra crispy bacon, bake the strips on a wire rack set over a baking sheet to allow the fat to drip away.

• Adjust the baking time based on the thickness of your bacon slices. Thinner slices may cook faster.

• You can also cook the bacon in a skillet over medium heat, flipping occasionally, until crispy.

• Store any leftover bacon strips in an airtight container in the refrigerator for up to 1 week.

94. Sausage bites

Ingredient:

- 1 lb Italian sausage, casings removed
- 1 tbsp olive oil
- 1 tsp dried oregano
- 1/2 tsp garlic powder
- 1/4 tsp red pepper flakes (optional, for spicy sausage)
- 1/4 tsp salt
- 1/4 tsp black pepper

Instructions:

1. Preheat your oven to 400°F (200°C). Line a baking sheet with parchment paper.

2. In a large bowl, combine the Italian sausage, olive oil, dried oregano, garlic powder, red pepper flakes (if using), salt, and black pepper. Mix well until the seasonings are evenly distributed.

3. Scoop the seasoned sausage mixture by the tablespoonful and roll them into small, bite•sized balls, about 1•inch in diameter.

4. Arrange the sausage bites in a single layer on the prepared baking sheet.

5. Bake the sausage bites in the preheated oven for 12•15 minutes, or until they are cooked through and lightly browned.

6. Remove the sausage bites from the oven and let them cool for a few minutes before serving.

Serve the sausage bites warm, as an appetizer or snack. They can be enjoyed on their own or with your favorite dipping sauces, such as barbecue sauce, honey mustard, or ranch dressing.

Tips:
- Use a high•quality Italian sausage for the best flavor.
- Adjust the amount of red pepper flakes based on your desired level of spiciness.
- You can also cook the sausage bites in a skillet over medium heat, turning occasionally, until they are cooked through.
- Store any leftover sausage bites in an airtight container in the refrigerator for up to 3 days.

95. Cheese cubes

Ingredient:

- 8 oz block of cheddar cheese, cut into 1•inch cubes
- 1 tbsp olive oil
- 1 tsp garlic powder
- 1 tsp dried oregano
- 1/2 tsp paprika
- 1/4 tsp salt

Instructions:

1. Preheat your oven to 400°F (200°C). Line a baking sheet with parchment paper.

2. In a medium bowl, combine the cubed cheddar cheese, olive oil, garlic powder, dried oregano, paprika, and salt. Toss gently to coat the cheese cubes evenly.

3. Spread the seasoned cheese cubes in a single layer on the prepared baking sheet.

4. Bake the cheese cubes in the preheated oven for 10•12 minutes, or until they are lightly golden brown and slightly crispy on the outside.

5. Remove the baked cheese cubes from the oven and let them cool for 5 minutes before serving.

Serve the baked cheese cubes warm, as a snack or appetizer. They can be enjoyed on their own or with crackers, bread, or your favorite dipping sauce.

Tips:
- Use a firm, flavorful cheese like cheddar, Parmesan, or Gouda for best results.

- Adjust the baking time based on the size of your cheese cubes. Smaller cubes may cook faster.

- For extra flavor, you can experiment with different seasoning blends, such as Italian seasoning, ranch seasoning, or Cajun spice mix.

- Store any leftover baked cheese cubes in an airtight container in the refrigerator for up to 5 days.

96. Tuna salad (without vegetables)

Ingredient:

- 2 (5 oz) cans tuna, drained
- 1/4 cup mayonnaise
- 1 tbsp lemon juice
- 1/4 tsp salt
- 1/8 tsp black pepper

Instructions:

1. In a medium bowl, combine the drained tuna, mayonnaise, lemon juice, salt, and black pepper. Mix well until fully incorporated.

2. Taste and adjust seasoning as needed, adding more mayonnaise for a creamier texture or more lemon juice for tanginess.

3. Serve the tuna salad on bread, crackers, or lettuce leaves. It also makes a great sandwich filling.

4. Store any leftover tuna salad in an airtight container in the refrigerator for up to 3-4 days.

That's it! This basic tuna salad recipe is quick and easy to make. You can customize it further by adding chopped hard-boiled eggs, relish, or other seasonings if desired. Enjoy!

97. Sardines in olive oil

Ingredient:

- 1 (4.25 oz) can of sardines in olive oil
- 1 tbsp fresh lemon juice
- 1 tsp chopped fresh parsley
- 1/4 tsp crushed red pepper flakes (optional)
- Salt and black pepper to taste

Instructions:

1. Drain the sardines from the can, reserving the olive oil.

2. In a small bowl, gently mix the drained sardines with the lemon juice, chopped parsley, and crushed red pepper flakes (if using). Season with salt and black pepper to taste.

3. Drizzle the reserved olive oil from the can over the sardine mixture and toss to coat.

4. Serve the sardines in olive oil immediately, or refrigerate for up to 3 days.

Serving Suggestions:
- Serve the sardines on top of crackers, toasted bread, or crostini.
- Use the sardines as a topping for salads or mixed greens.
- Enjoy the sardines as a snack on their own, with a squeeze of lemon juice.
- Mix the sardines into pasta dishes, rice bowls, or omelets.

Tips:
- Look for high•quality, sustainably•sourced sardines packed in olive oil.
- Adjust the amount of lemon juice, parsley, and red pepper flakes to suit your taste preferences.
- The olive oil from the can can be used for cooking or drizzling over the sardines.
- Refrigerate any leftover sardines in the reserved olive oil for up to 3 days.

98. Deviled eggs

Ingredient:

- 12 hard•boiled eggs
- 1/4 cup mayonnaise
- 1 tbsp Dijon mustard
- 1 tsp white vinegar or lemon juice
- 1/4 tsp salt
- 1/8 tsp black pepper
- Paprika for garnish (optional)

Instructions:

1. Peel the hard•boiled eggs and cut them in half lengthwise.

2. Carefully scoop out the yolks and place them in a medium bowl.

3. Add the mayonnaise, Dijon mustard, vinegar or lemon juice, salt, and black pepper to the yolks. Mash and mix everything together until smooth and creamy.

4. Using a spoon or piping bag, fill the egg white halves evenly with the yolk mixture.

5. Sprinkle the tops of the filled eggs lightly with paprika, if desired.

6. Refrigerate the deviled eggs for at least 30 minutes before serving to allow the flavors to meld.

Tips:
- For extra flavor, you can add a small amount of finely chopped onion, pickle relish, or a dash of hot sauce to the yolk mixture.

- Garnish the deviled eggs with a sprinkle of chopped chives, crumbled bacon, or a small piece of pickle.

- Make ahead and refrigerate for up to 3 days in an airtight container.

Deviled eggs are a classic appetizer or side dish that are easy to make and always a crowd•pleaser. Enjoy!

99. Salami slices

Ingredient:

• 8•10 oz salami, thinly sliced

That's it! Just the salami slices.

Instructions:

1. Arrange the thinly sliced salami on a serving platter or plate.

2. You can leave the slices as•is, or you can fold or roll them up for a more decorative presentation.

Serving Suggestions:

• Serve the salami slices as part of a charcuterie board or appetizer platter, along with other cured meats, cheeses, olives, crackers, etc.

• Use the salami slices to make mini sandwiches or wraps. Layer them with cheese, pickles, mustard, etc.

• Drizzle the salami slices with a bit of olive oil and sprinkle with freshly cracked black pepper.

• Arrange the salami slices in a spiral or overlapping pattern on a plate for a simple yet elegant presentation.

• Pair the salami with toasted bread, crackers, or crostini for dipping in olive oil or balsamic vinegar.

The key is to use high•quality, thinly sliced salami for the best flavor and texture. Enjoy the salty, savory goodness of these simple salami slices!

100. Prosciutto•wrapped cheese

Ingredient:

• 8 oz block of cheese (such as cheddar, gouda, or brie)
• 4•6 slices of prosciutto
• Toothpicks or skewers (optional)

Instructions:

1. Cut the block of cheese into 1•inch cubes or wedges, depending on the shape of the cheese.

2. Wrap each piece of cheese tightly with a slice of prosciutto, overlapping the edges slightly to fully encase the cheese.

3. If desired, secure the prosciutto•wrapped cheese with a toothpick or small skewer.

4. Arrange the prosciutto•wrapped cheese on a serving platter.

5. Serve immediately or refrigerate until ready to serve.

Tips:
• Choose a firm, semi•soft cheese that will hold its shape when wrapped in prosciutto.

• For a more decorative presentation, you can use longer slices of prosciutto and wrap them around the cheese in a spiral pattern.

• Serve the prosciutto•wrapped cheese with crackers, bread, olives, or other charcuterie items.

• This makes a great easy appetizer or snack.

Enjoy the salty, savory combination of the prosciutto and creamy cheese!

101. Meatballs

Ingredient:

- 1 lb ground beef (or a mix of ground beef and ground pork)
- 1 cup breadcrumbs
- 1/2 cup milk
- 1 egg
- 1/4 cup grated Parmesan cheese
- 2 cloves garlic, minced
- 1 tsp dried oregano
- 1 tsp salt
- 1/2 tsp black pepper

Instructions:

1. In a large bowl, combine the ground beef, breadcrumbs, milk, egg, Parmesan, garlic, oregano, salt, and pepper. Mix gently with your hands until just combined, being careful not to overmix.

2. Scoop out heaping tablespoon•sized portions of the meat mixture and roll them into round balls, about 1•1.5 inches in diameter.

3. In a large skillet or Dutch oven, heat 2•3 tablespoons of olive oil over medium•high heat.

4. Working in batches, add the meatballs to the hot oil and cook, turning occasionally, until browned on all sides, about 5•7 minutes per batch.

5. Transfer the cooked meatballs to a paper towel•lined plate.

6. Once all the meatballs are cooked, you can serve them as•is, or add them to a sauce (such as marinara or Swedish meatball sauce) and simmer for 10•15 minutes to allow the flavors to meld.

Tips:
- For extra•tender meatballs, soak the breadcrumbs in the milk for 5•10 minutes before mixing.
- You can bake the meatballs in the oven at 400°F for 15•20 minutes instead of frying.
- Try adding finely chopped onion, parsley, or other herbs to the meatball mixture.

Enjoy these classic, versatile homemade meatballs!

102. Canned mackerel

Ingredient:

- 2 (4.25 oz) cans of mackerel, drained and flaked
- 2 tablespoons mayonnaise
- 1 tablespoon Dijon mustard
- 1 tablespoon lemon juice
- 1 teaspoon finely chopped dill (or 1/2 tsp dried dill)
- 1/4 cup finely diced celery
- 2 tablespoons finely diced red onion
- Salt and pepper to taste

Instructions:

1. In a medium bowl, combine the flaked mackerel, mayonnaise, Dijon mustard, lemon juice, and dill. Mix well until the mackerel is evenly coated.

2. Fold in the diced celery and red onion. Season with salt and pepper to taste.

3. Cover and refrigerate the mackerel salad for at least 30 minutes to allow the flavors to meld.

Serving Suggestions:
- Serve the mackerel salad on top of mixed greens or lettuce leaves for a light salad.
- Scoop the salad onto crackers, toasted bread, or cucumber slices for an easy appetizer.
- Mix the mackerel salad with cooked pasta for a heartier main dish.
- Use the salad as a filling for sandwiches or wraps.

Tips:
- For a creamier texture, add an extra tablespoon of mayonnaise.
- Customize the salad by adding chopped hard-boiled eggs, diced pickles, or capers.
- Substitute Greek yogurt for some or all of the mayonnaise for a tangier flavor.
- Store the mackerel salad in an airtight container in the refrigerator for up to 3 days.

Enjoy this flavorful and protein-packed mackerel salad!

103. Roast beef slices

Ingredient:

• 8•10 oz thinly sliced roast beef

That's it! Just the roast beef slices.

Instructions:

1. Arrange the thinly sliced roast beef on a serving platter or plate.

2. You can leave the slices as•is, or you can fold or roll them up for a more decorative presentation.

Serving Suggestions:

• Serve the roast beef slices as part of a sandwich or wrap. Layer them with cheese, lettuce, tomato, onion, etc.

• Use the roast beef slices to make mini sandwiches or appetizers. Top them with a small slice of cheese, a pickle, or a dollop of horseradish sauce.

• Arrange the roast beef slices on a charcuterie board or appetizer platter, along with other cured meats, cheeses, olives, crackers, etc.

• Drizzle the roast beef slices with a bit of au jus or horseradish sauce for extra flavor.

• Sprinkle the roast beef slices with freshly cracked black pepper or a seasoning blend.

• Serve the roast beef slices at room temperature or slightly chilled.

The key is to use high•quality, thinly sliced roast beef for the best texture and flavor. Enjoy these simple yet delicious roast beef slices!

104. Liverwurst

Ingredient:

• 8•10 oz liverwurst, sliced

That's it! Just the liverwurst slices.

Instructions:

1. Slice the liverwurst into 1/4•inch thick pieces.

2. Arrange the liverwurst slices on a serving platter or plate.

Serving Suggestions:

• Serve the liverwurst slices on crackers, bread, or toast points. Top with thinly sliced onion, pickles, or mustard.

• Use the liverwurst slices to make mini sandwiches or appetizers. Layer them with cheese, lettuce, tomato, etc.

• Arrange the liverwurst slices on a charcuterie board or appetizer platter, along with other cured meats, cheeses, olives, and accompaniments.

• Spread the liverwurst onto celery sticks or cucumber slices for a low•carb snack.

• Top the liverwurst slices with a dollop of whole grain mustard or a drizzle of olive oil and balsamic vinegar.

• Serve the liverwurst at room temperature or slightly chilled.

Tips:
• Choose a high•quality, flavorful liverwurst for the best taste.
• Experiment with different types of liverwurst, such as chicken or pork.
• Garnish the liverwurst slices with fresh herbs, capers, or a sprinkle of paprika for added color and flavor.

Liverwurst has a rich, savory flavor that pairs well with a variety of accompaniments. Enjoy these simple liverwurst slices as a tasty snack or appetizer.

105. Fried pork skins

Ingredient:

- 1 lb pork skin, cut into 1·inch pieces
- Vegetable or peanut oil for frying
- Salt

Instructions:

1. Rinse the pork skin pieces under cold water and pat them completely dry with paper towels. This is important to get them as dry as possible before frying.

2. In a large heavy·bottomed pot or Dutch oven, heat 2·3 inches of oil to 350°F. Use a deep·fry or candy thermometer to monitor the temperature.

3. Working in batches, carefully add the pork skin pieces to the hot oil. Fry for 5·7 minutes, turning occasionally, until golden brown and crispy.

4. Use a slotted spoon or tongs to transfer the fried pork skins to a paper towel·lined plate or baking sheet.

5. Immediately season the hot pork skins generously with salt.

6. Allow the oil to return to temperature between batches. Avoid overcrowding the pot.

7. Serve the crispy fried pork skins warm. They make a great snack or appetizer.

Tips:
- For extra crispiness, you can par·boil the pork skin pieces for 5·10 minutes before patting them dry and frying.
- Experiment with different seasoning blends, such as chili powder, garlic powder, or Cajun spice.
- Store any leftover fried pork skins in an airtight container at room temperature for up to 3 days.

Enjoy these crunchy, salty fried pork skins! They're a delicious and addictive snack.

106. Smoked sausages

Ingredient:

- 3 lbs ground pork (or a mix of pork and beef)
- 2 tsp salt
- 1 tsp black pepper
- 1 tsp garlic powder
- 1 tsp smoked paprika
- 1/2 tsp cayenne pepper (optional for spicy)
- Sausage casings (natural or synthetic)

Instructions:

1. In a large bowl, combine the ground pork, salt, black pepper, garlic powder, smoked paprika, and cayenne (if using). Mix well until the seasonings are evenly distributed.

2. Stuff the seasoned pork mixture into sausage casings, making 4·6 inch links. Twist or tie off the casings between each link.

3. Preheat your smoker to 225°F. If you don't have a smoker, you can use a charcoal or gas grill set up for indirect heat.

4. Place the sausage links directly on the grill grates or smoker racks, making sure they are not touching.

5. Smoke the sausages for 2·3 hours, or until they reach an internal temperature of 160°F. Add wood chips or chunks to the smoker as needed to maintain a steady smoke.

6. Once fully cooked, remove the sausages from the smoker and let them rest for 5·10 minutes before serving.

7. Serve the smoked sausages hot, or let them cool completely before storing in the refrigerator for up to 1 week.

Tips:
- For extra flavor, you can add other dried herbs and spices like fennel, thyme, or red pepper flakes.
- Try using a combination of pork and beef, or even venison, for the ground meat.
- Experiment with different types of wood chips, like apple, hickory, or mesquite, to impart different smoky flavors.

107. Beef sticks

Ingredient:

- 2 lbs ground beef
- 2 tsp salt
- 1 tsp black pepper
- 1 tsp garlic powder
- 1 tsp onion powder
- 1 tsp smoked paprika
- 1/2 tsp red pepper flakes (optional for spicy)
- Casings (optional)

Instructions:

1. In a large bowl, combine the ground beef, salt, black pepper, garlic powder, onion powder, smoked paprika, and red pepper flakes (if using). Mix well until the seasonings are evenly distributed.

2. If using casings, stuff the seasoned ground beef into the casings, making sure to pack it in tightly. Twist or tie off the casings into 4•6 inch links.

3. If not using casings, you can shape the seasoned ground beef into long, thin sticks or logs, about 4•6 inches long.

4. Place the beef sticks on a parchment•lined baking sheet or dehydrator trays.

5. Dehydrate the beef sticks at 155°F for 4•6 hours, or until they reach your desired dryness and chewiness. Alternatively, you can bake them in the oven at 200°F for 2•3 hours.

6. Once fully dried, let the beef sticks cool completely before handling.

7. Store the beef sticks in an airtight container at room temperature for up to 2 weeks.

Tips:
- For extra flavor, you can add other dried herbs and spices like paprika, cayenne, or cumin.
- Experiment with different types of ground meat, like turkey or venison, for variety.
- Slice the dried beef sticks diagonally for a more uniform shape.

Enjoy these homemade beef sticks as a protein•packed snack or on•the•go treat!

108. Anchovies

Ingredient:

• 1 (2 oz) tin of anchovies in oil

That's it! Just the tin of anchovies.

Instructions:

1. Open the tin of anchovies and drain off any excess oil, if desired.

2. Arrange the anchovies on a small plate or platter. You can leave them whole or gently separate them into individual fillets.

Serving Suggestions:

• Serve the anchovies as part of a charcuterie board or appetizer platter, along with other cured meats, cheeses, olives, crackers, etc.

• Top bruschetta or crostini with the anchovies for a salty, savory bite.

• Mix the anchovies into a Caesar salad dressing for extra flavor.

• Use the anchovies to top pizza, pasta dishes, or roasted vegetables.

• Mash the anchovies into butter to make an anchovy compound butter.

• Wrap the anchovies around olives, capers, or cornichons for a quick and easy hors d'oeuvre.

The key is to use high•quality, jarred or canned anchovies packed in oil. Anchovies have a strong, salty, umami flavor that pairs well with many other ingredients. Enjoy them as a simple, protein•packed snack or as an ingredient to enhance other dishes.

109. Roasted bone marrow

Ingredient:

- 4•6 beef marrow bones, about 3•4 inches long
- Coarse sea salt
- Freshly cracked black pepper
- Lemon wedges, for serving
- Crusty bread, for serving

Instructions:

1. Preheat your oven to 400°F (200°C).

2. Rinse the marrow bones under cold water and pat them dry thoroughly with paper towels. This will help them roast properly.

3. Place the marrow bones upright in a baking dish or on a rimmed baking sheet. Make sure they are standing up straight and not touching each other.

4. Generously season the exposed marrow with coarse sea salt and freshly cracked black pepper.

5. Roast the marrow bones in the preheated oven for 15•20 minutes, or until the marrow is soft and starting to ooze out of the bones.

6. Remove the roasted marrow bones from the oven and let them cool for 5 minutes.

7. Use a small spoon or fork to scoop the soft, creamy marrow out of the bones and onto a plate or board.

8. Serve the roasted bone marrow immediately, with lemon wedges and crusty bread for dipping.

Tips:
- For best flavor, use high•quality, fresh beef marrow bones.
- You can add other seasonings like garlic, herbs, or a drizzle of olive oil to the marrow.
- Serve the roasted bone marrow as an appetizer or alongside a steak or other hearty main dish.
- Leftovers can be refrigerated for up to 3 days and reheated gently before serving.

110. Biltong

Ingredient:

- 2 lbs beef sirloin or top round, cut into long, thin strips about 1/4 inch thick
- 1/4 cup brown vinegar
- 2 tbsp coarse salt
- 2 tsp ground coriander
- 1 tsp black pepper
- 1 tsp brown sugar
- 1 tsp garlic powder

Instructions:

1. In a large bowl, combine the vinegar, salt, coriander, black pepper, brown sugar, and garlic powder. Add the beef strips and toss to coat evenly.

2. Cover the bowl and refrigerate for 12•24 hours, turning the beef occasionally to ensure even marinating.

3. Remove the marinated beef from the fridge and pat the strips dry with paper towels.

4. Hang the beef strips or place them on a biltong hanging rack in a cool, dry, well•ventilated area. The ideal temperature is 60•70°F with low humidity.

5. Allow the biltong to dry for 3•5 days, depending on the thickness of the strips and your desired level of dryness. The biltong should become firm and leathery when ready.

6. Once dried, store the biltong in an airtight container at room temperature for up to 2 weeks.

Tips:
- For best results, use a fan to circulate the air around the drying biltong.
- You can also dry the biltong in a dehydrator set to 155°F for 6•12 hours.
- Experiment with different spice blends, such as adding chili powder or curry powder.
- Slice the biltong across the grain for a more tender texture.

Enjoy this classic South African dried meat snack! Biltong is high in protein and makes a great on•the•go treat.

111. Grilled chicken strips

Ingredient:

- 1 lb boneless, skinless chicken breasts, cut into 1·inch thick strips
- 2 tbsp olive oil
- 1 tsp garlic powder
- 1 tsp paprika
- 1 tsp dried oregano
- 1/2 tsp salt
- 1/4 tsp black pepper

Instructions:

1. In a large bowl, combine the chicken strips, olive oil, garlic powder, paprika, oregano, salt, and black pepper. Toss to coat the chicken evenly.

2. Preheat your grill or grill pan to medium·high heat.

3. Thread the seasoned chicken strips onto metal or wooden skewers, leaving a little space between each piece.

4. Grill the chicken skewers for 3·4 minutes per side, or until the chicken is cooked through and reaches an internal temperature of 165°F.

5. Remove the grilled chicken strips from the skewers and serve immediately.

Serving Suggestions:

- Serve the grilled chicken strips as an appetizer or main dish, with your choice of dipping sauces like ranch, barbecue, or honey mustard.

- Use the grilled chicken strips in salads, wraps, or as a topping for pizzas or pasta dishes.

- For extra flavor, you can marinate the chicken in a mixture of olive oil, lemon juice, and herbs for 30 minutes to 1 hour before grilling.

- Try different seasoning blends, such as Cajun, lemon·pepper, or Italian herbs.

112. Greek yogurt (plain, no sugar)

Ingredient:

• 1 quart (4 cups) whole milk
• 1/4 cup plain yogurt with active cultures

Instructions:

1. In a large saucepan, heat the milk over medium heat, stirring occasionally, until it reaches 180•190°F. This will take around 10•15 minutes.

2. Remove the saucepan from the heat and let the milk cool down to 110•115°F. This will take about 30 minutes.

3. Once the milk has cooled to the proper temperature, stir in the 1/4 cup of plain yogurt with active cultures. Make sure to incorporate it well.

4. Pour the yogurt mixture into a clean container, cover, and let it incubate at 110°F for 6•8 hours. This allows the yogurt cultures to ferment and thicken the yogurt.

5. After the incubation period, refrigerate the yogurt for at least 4 hours, or until completely chilled.

6. Once chilled, the plain Greek yogurt is ready to enjoy! It will have a thick, creamy texture.

Tips:
• Use whole milk for the richest, creamiest yogurt. You can also use 2% or nonfat milk.
• Make sure to use a plain yogurt with live, active cultures to act as the starter.
• Incubate the yogurt in a warm oven, slow cooker, or yogurt maker for best results.
• Strain the yogurt through a cheesecloth or coffee filter to make it even thicker, if desired.
• Store the plain Greek yogurt in an airtight container in the refrigerator for up to 1 week.

Enjoy this simple, protein•packed plain Greek yogurt on its own or use it in recipes!

113. Cottage cheese

Ingredient:

• 1 gallon (4 quarts) whole milk
• 1 cup buttermilk
• 1 tsp salt

Instructions:

1. In a large pot, heat the milk over medium heat, stirring occasionally, until it reaches 185•195°F. This will take around 15•20 minutes.

2. Remove the pot from the heat and stir in the buttermilk. The milk should start to curdle and separate into curds and whey.

3. Cover the pot and let it sit undisturbed for 30 minutes to 1 hour, until the curds have fully formed and the whey has separated.

4. Line a colander with cheesecloth or a clean kitchen towel. Carefully pour the curds and whey mixture through the colander, allowing the whey to drain off.

5. Gently transfer the curds to a clean bowl. Sprinkle the salt over the curds and stir to combine.

6. For a smoother texture, you can lightly press the curds with the back of a spoon to release more whey.

7. Refrigerate the cottage cheese for at least 2 hours before serving to allow the flavors to meld.

Tips:
• Use whole milk for the richest, creamiest cottage cheese.
• Adjust the salt to your taste preference.
• For a drier, more crumbly cottage cheese, let the curds drain for longer.
• Experiment with adding herbs, spices, or fruit to the cottage cheese.
• Store the cottage cheese in an airtight container in the refrigerator for up to 1 week.

Enjoy this homemade, fresh cottage cheese on its own or use it in recipes like lasagna, dips, or as a protein•packed snack.

*Congratulations on completing the **"Carnivore Diet Cookbook for Seniors: Transform Your Diet with Protein-Rich, Senior-Friendly Recipes."** We hope this culinary journey has been as enriching for you as it has been for us to create. By exploring the diverse and delicious recipes within these pages, you've taken significant steps toward optimizing your health and well-being through a nutrient-dense, meat-focused diet.*

Transitioning to a carnivore diet can be a transformative experience, especially for seniors looking to enhance their vitality and overall quality of life. The recipes provided in this book are designed to not only satisfy your taste buds but also to ensure that your body receives the essential nutrients it needs to thrive. From improving muscle mass and bone density to boosting energy levels and cognitive function, the benefits of a protein-rich diet are profound.

As you continue to incorporate these recipes into your daily routine, remember that the journey to better health is ongoing. Listening to your body and making mindful dietary choices are key to sustaining the positive changes you've achieved. Feel free to revisit your favorite recipes and experiment with new ones, tailoring your meals to suit your personal preferences and nutritional needs.

We also encourage you to share your newfound knowledge and culinary creations with family and friends. By doing so, you can inspire others to explore the benefits of the carnivore diet and enjoy the same delicious, health-boosting meals.

Thank you for allowing us to be a part of your health journey. We hope that this cookbook has provided you with valuable insights, practical tips, and a collection of mouthwatering recipes that will continue to support your well-being for years to come. Here's to a future filled with health, happiness, and the joys of delicious, protein-rich meals!

Wishing you all the best on your journey to optimal health and vitality.

Bon appétit!

9 798328 562249